Clothes The Deal

Clothes
The
Deal

THE GUIDE *for* TRANSFORMATIVE PERSONAL STYLE

JENN MAPP BRESSAN

NEW YORK

LONDON • NASHVILLE • MELBOURNE • VANCOUVER

Clothes The Deal

THE GUIDE for TRANSFORMATIVE PERSONAL STYLE

© 2019 JENN MAPP BRESSAN

Published in New York, New York, by Morgan James Publishing in partnership with Difference Press. Morgan James is a trademark of Morgan James, LLC. www.MorganJamesPublishing.com

ISBN 978-1-64279-260-7 paperback
ISBN 978-1-64279-261-4 eBook
Library of Congress Control Number: 2018910661

Cover Design by:
Rachel Lopez
www.r2cdesign.com

Interior Design by:
Bonnie Bushman
The Whole Caboodle Graphic Design

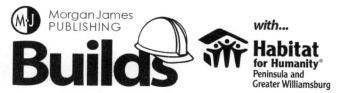

In an effort to support local communities, raise awareness and funds, Morgan James Publishing donates a percentage of all book sales for the life of each book to Habitat for Humanity Peninsula and Greater Williamsburg.

Get involved today! Visit
www.MorganJamesBuilds.com

Dedication

For my Aunt Catherine, who taught me to dress like myself,
stand in my truth and walk like a New Yorker.

Table of Contents

Foreword

When I first met Jenn, she and I both worked for Ann Ratner, the terminally fabulous founder of Washington, DC based Bubbles Hair Salons. At 14 years old, I landed my first real job as a shampoo tech in the Bubbles Annapolis Mall location. Around the same time, Ann hired Jenn to develop her Cibu brand of haircare products. Jenn spent a lot of time in our salon facilitating education, hosting events, and promoting Cibu. My first impression of Jenn was of an excited, fabulous, and hyper-focused mini Ann Ratner. Jenn couldn't have been more than 24 years old (which was still pretty old to me) but even at an age when most young people are testing the limits of appropriate office attire, her look was always on point—sleek, authentic, creative. She owned it. This girl was determined to make Cibu a *thing*—and she dressed for the part. It was no surprise to me that she took Cibu from an in-house haircare line to headlining sponsor of my first New York Fashion Week show in less than three years.

The idea that our appearance shapes our reality is inherent to my design philosophy. Since day one, I've been passionate about democratizing style—I firmly believe every woman, of every age, color, and size should be able to put on a dress and feel like she can conquer the world.

I also recognize that style isn't a natural reflex for everyone. It takes energy and intention to feel fantastic in your skin. A huge part of the challenge is conquering closet chaos—so many women wake up every day and confront a wardrobe that doesn't love them back. Imagine how much more stylish they would feel if their closets were filled only with garments that made them feel fantastic?

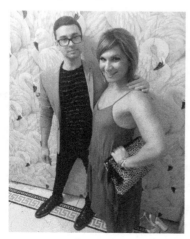

Jenn and Christian at his boutique The Curated NYC, September 2018.

Personal style isn't reserved for the rich or connected. Personal style comes from dressing with authenticity and loving yourself enough to make the effort. This is the core philosophy of *Clothes the Deal* and the reason I wanted to endorse Jenn's book—with the right tools and the right intentions, you can feel fantastic in your own skin. And you deserve to feel fantastic.

Both Jenn and I started our careers in the salon world—we understand the power of simple changes. We're also both real life examples of the transformative power of personal style. When you show up looking like a boss—you're going to leave with the job.

Christian Siriano

Introduction

"I do think women can have it all… Our life comes in segments, and we have to understand that we can have it all if we're not trying to do it all at once."
—Madeleine Albright

This book is not written by a famous Hollywood stylist, it is not a buying guide intended to replace your entire wardrobe, this is not a tip sheet to 10x your social following by dressing like an influencer. This is an exercise in personal style for you—the woman who "has it all." Head of her class, self-made entrepreneur, senior partner, life coach, therapist, fitness guru. You are every ambitious junior associate's American dream—the powerful, educated, accomplished businesswoman with all the accolades and a salary to match.

So why can't you dress like it?

Cut yourself some slack, you were never that into fashion anyway. Sure, you appreciate a well-dressed woman and can recognize chic when you see it, but putting outfits together? Not your thing. You had a career to craft, kids to raise, a mortgage, and a husband. So why now? Let me guess. Life caught up with you. When you entered the work force, women in your profession dressed a certain way (like men in skirts, amiright?) but fast forward to 2018 and these younger associates—*your* direct reports, well they have a different vibe. They aren't attached to traditional notions of appropriate workplace attire and it works for them. Now, when you see your reflection in the elevator door, your eyes are drawn to your ill-fitting jacket, dated pants, and tired eyes. It's painfully apparent that your outdated look is overshadowing your achievements and if you don't do something to refresh it soon, you may lose all the credibility you worked so hard to earn.

The good news? You are so smart and I know a thing or two about the power of the right outfit. I am going to teach you that personal style is a skill set you can master. My goal is not to give you a magical makeover or dress you like Angelina Jolie (humanitarian Angie, not blood vial), my goal is to show you how chucking 70 percent of your clothes can make you look 100 percent more stylish. We will unpack all the reasons you are clinging to clothes that do not serve you and devise a strategy to curb late night "on-wine" shopping once and for all. We will examine what works for you and what doesn't and we will fill in the gaps with the *right* clothes: clothes that fit, flatter, and command authority. Signature garments that just feel like you.

Once you have a working wardrobe I will teach you a simple Four-Step Formula guaranteed to inspire countless outfit variations so you will always have something to wear—from staff meeting to client cocktails to weekends with kids to your next hot date. At the end of this book, you will have the formula to feel put together and proud of your appearance every single day—and change your life in the process. This book is about evolving into the best version of yourself so you can stop thinking about what you look like and get back to being the boss.

My Story

As far back as I can remember, I've had a passion for fashion. In fifth grade, after watching Grease, I became obsessed with poodle skirts. In 1987, you couldn't just pluck one from the costume selection off Amazon—I had to be resourceful. So, I gathered every skirt in my closet and layered them one on top of the other until I achieved what I considered crinoline-worthy girth. My Peter-Pan-collared St. Pius X uniform blouse topped off the look perfectly. Bless my mother's heart, she never blinked an eye. That afternoon we went to TJ Maxx and a middle-aged lady in the blouse aisle eyed me up and down with a confused smirk. Only then did it occur to me I might look ridiculous. No matter.

In eighth grade, I went way into athleisure, which in 1990, consisted of very bright sneakers and baggy jeans worn inside out. Thankfully I wore a uniform to school so the jeans were a non-issue but the shoes! Oh, I had to have those shoes. My father was not compliant. In an act of desperation, I landed a newspaper route. Within weeks, the red suede Champion high tops were mine. Followed by another pair and another until the breadth of my suede Etonic collection was the envy of the middle school circuit. This was very satisfying.

This mindset continued through high school, college, and into adulthood—clothes were my craft. I was this person or that person, never attached to the same look for long and forever devising ways to hack, sew, thrift, or gift my way into a fresh new outfit. When I didn't have money, I scoured consignment stores and eBay or I waited tables to support my love of outfit crafting.

At 24, with no marketing experience, I landed the job that would launch my branding career. My boss Ann, a dynamic hairdresser turned salon tycoon, was a firecracker and terminally chic. I'll never forget my first interview. She was wearing these sublime Chanel eyeglasses—transparent frames with what I would later learn were detachable arms so she could swap colors on a whim. I wanted nothing but to be just like her, both in income and wardrobe. Once on a plane, Ann was reading a fashion magazine, mindlessly flipping a suede pump on and off her heel. Manolo Blahniks, I observed. She looked up at me and pointed to a pair of shoes on the page. "$765!" she exclaimed. "Who would pay that much for shoes?" I looked at the page. Manolo Blahniks. I vowed to reach a point when I didn't even realize how much I paid for my shoes.

By the time I turned 30, the hair care line I created for Ann's salons was taking off. I traveled up and down the east coast to visit salons supporting our brand. Almost all of our locations were inside of malls. Every off minute was spent shopping for *mini-Ann* outfits. Christian Louboutin simple pumps, Fendi work tote, Georgio Armani silk camisole, Theory blazer, Vince cashmere, Gucci bikini, and more than a few pairs of Manolo Blahniks. Every designer acquisition sparked a sense of accomplishment and a boat load of joy.

And then life happened. I got married, he started a business, and it failed. At work, newly hired executives "stabilized my income." We had our first child. We bought a starter home—inside the Beltway (DC speak for small and expensive). I got pregnant again and after our daughter was born, our new house quickly became way too small. During this time our disposable income tightened, my responsibilities and focus pivoted, and I gained and lost two pregnancies worth of weight—buying clothes the entire time in cadence with my mood.

Six months after Ashby was born, I was back at work full time, nursing all night, pumping all-day, and sleeping practically never. I returned from maternity leave to find most of my responsibilities had been delegated. I was sleep-deprived, with an infant, a two-year-old, and a career that suddenly made me feel like garbage. Our 1000 sq. ft. house vibrated at chaos level and now we (read: I) had to stage it to sell.

While planning the logistics for our move, I was confronted with a real problem—the new house was bigger but the closets were definitely not. To accommodate my massive wardrobe (stuffed with ten years of Ann-inspired business separates, maternity clothes for two pregnancies in two different seasons, and all the ill-fitting, random crap I bought online at 3 a.m. while nursing) I had installed an Elfa closet system that took up the entire wall of our laundry room. There was no such solution in the new house.

As I looked at my dense collection of clothes (many with tags, many expensive, most unworn) I felt shame, guilt, overwhelm, and panic. Not one drop of joy. My wardrobe, once a source of pride and accomplishment, was no more serving my mind state than the piles of unfolded laundry in baskets all over our house.

I took to Pinterest to unearth some magical organization system and instead I found the photo that changed my life. It was of a reach-in closet that looked more like a garment rack at a photo shoot than any wardrobe in my house. It was elegantly sparse, populated with around 25 coordinating garments, all minimal in their aesthetic. Everything about this picture spoke to me. I was enchanted by its scarcity and the sense of calm it generated in my heart chakra. The actual clothes reflected my fantasy postnatal work style (sleek, minimalist, versatile, comfortable). I also realized that rack contained roughly 10 percent of the 300+ garments in my current wardrobe—and exactly the amount of my wardrobe I actually wore. Clicking the link on the picture, I discovered an article about capsule wardrobes.

Apparently, there was an entire movement centered on giving away most of your clothes to create a seasonal capsule of garments that mixed and matched and that you actually wore. Supposedly, the process was cathartic and powerful and could make you feel like you were actually in control of your life.

Sold!

The next day I ruthlessly ripped through my wardrobe, using only my intuition to guide the process. If I had even one millisecond of hesitation about a garment—to the purge pile it went. What surprised me was how ready I was to let go of my imaginary rich career girl story and embrace the reality of now. It took me two months to get rid of all of those clothes, but I did it and regretted not one castaway DVF dress.

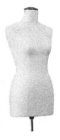

Chapter One

The ROI of Personal Style

*"Dress shabbily and they remember the dress; dress
impeccably and they remember the woman."*
—Coco Chanel

The New Face of Business

Fifteen years ago, in 2001, a much-referenced consumer research
study conducted by firm Yankelovich Partners, Inc., titled "Work
Your Image: The Importance of Appearance on the Job" reported
that 76 percent of respondents believe that a woman's appearance
affects whether she is taken seriously, asked to participate in meetings
with upper management, or is well regarded by colleagues and
supervisors. Sixty-four percent believe that her appearance will lead
to consideration for raises or promotion.

Fast forward to 2018. Now you are upper management and the implications of your personal work style have evolved far beyond meeting participation. Executive, entrepreneur, or partner—if you have a marketing strategy, the pressure is on to get comfortable in the spotlight. Whether it requires you to be on camera, on stage, or contribute to digital campaigns, in our socially driven business world, content is king; like it or not, your years of experience make you the voice and face of that content. If you can't step into the role of brand ambassador and own it, you risk irrelevance.

Youth is Wasted on the Young

We've all heard the catch phrases "dress for success" or "dress for the job you want, not the job you have." So what if you already have the job? In your late 20s and 30s, when you were tending to your career, youth blurred the jagged edges of your style deficiency. Today your ill-fitted suit is amplified by tired eyes and way less shiny hair. There is hardly a day you feel great about the way you look and when you see yourself in the mirror, you don't see years of professional accolades, you see a tired middle-aged woman who looks frumpy and feels practically invisible. You are not alone.

My highest profile client is exactly the woman we'd assume "has it all." An award-winning journalist and news anchor, she has accolades, celebrity, a beautiful family, and a lovely home in a coveted neighborhood. To top it all off—she's tall, honey blonde, and gorgeous. Her closet was neat, with what I felt was an appropriate assortment of bright, quality garments for a woman on television every day. It took me a couple of sessions to noodle out what she actually needed. Turns out that she contacted me after a wave of personnel changes at her network. Until recently, she was the junior member of the news team but now, at 45, she was suddenly a veteran and the other gals … well, they were younger and they dressed in a way that made her feel old. She didn't want me to transform her style or dress her like a woman half her age, she just needed a fresh perspective—and it made all the difference.

Like my client, there has never been a more important time in your life than now to invest in an image refresh. Not just because study after study proves that what you wear matters; this change is imperative because how you dress has a direct effect on how *you* feel about yourself—and how you feel about yourself is directly related to your ability to generate revenue, manage a team, and represent your business in an increasingly visual world.

You Lead How You Think

A 2015 study published in *Scientific American* reinforces the idea our that clothing influences how others respond to us, but it goes a step further to argue that self-image also frames how we respond to the world at large. When we feel good about our appearance, we are more apt to perceive our environment through an empowered, "I'm-a-bada**-let's-do-this-thing!" lens. What happens next is simple law of attraction—our powerful self-talk begets powerful results.

What thoughts are you generating about your appearance every day? Are those thoughts manifesting a platform for heartfelt mentorship? Do they drive your creative process to deliver unprecedented work? Do those thoughts close leads—daily?

A woman who invests in her appearance knows that she looks good. A woman who knows she looks good leaves her house with a mindset primed to propel sales, projects, and life forward, every single day.

Whats Your Insecurity Style?

Consider for a minute how your self-image shapes your day-to-day work life. Do you enjoy open, warm, and friendly relationships with your direct reports? Do they feel empowered to ask for professional guidance or are they constantly talking to you about their personal lives? Do you feel comfortable traveling with colleagues? Have you embraced visual communication tools like Skype or would you rather hash out a project over e-mail than get on camera? Do you look forward to client dinners? Are you perceived as "cold?" Have you ever dismissed a younger or more stylish colleague's ideas because you have "feelings" about the way they look?

In my client work, which always begins with a radically transparent conversation about self-image and thought patterns, I've identified four distinct professional archetypes that capable women embody to compensate for a negative self-image:

Andrea would rather lose a lead than meet a client in person or on a video call. She works from home, executing virtual deliverables (graphic design, copy writing, editing, coding, journalism, calligraphy), and that suits her just fine. She has real talent and business savvy. Over the course of her career, she has collected a wealth of knowledge on her subject matter and what it takes to scale. Her actual closet doesn't hold many clothes, as the majority of her wardrobe is dresser material: a hodgepodge of LuLaRoe (she had a friend, ok?), yoga pants that have never seen the inside of a studio, and denim. Andrea recognizes she has an opportunity to coach, build a social digital presence, and attach a brand face to her powerful work but she's terrified to be seen.

Elsa is cold. At least that's what people say about her behind her back. She is highly educated, incredibly accomplished, and very, very sharp. Elsa doesn't do small talk. Her profession (lawyer, lobbyist, CEO, senior executive) requires her to be on her game at all times. She prefers to work with men. Her leadership style is authoritative and she'd rather hire people who know how to do the job than mentor them into a role. In her heart, Elsa craves connection but has all these hang ups from high school about not being pretty enough to attempt style. She spent her career building sales—and thick walls to defend herself from criticism. Her closet is large but sparsely populated and she's carried the same work horse briefcase for five years. Ever capable, had it not been for a personal crisis (divorce or death), Elsa would have never contacted me for help.

Sally is everyone's friend. She is warm, kind, and a little bit scattered. Colleagues talk to her about themselves all the time. Sally is an accomplished, yet non-threatening member of the executive team—incessantly positive, she always puts the needs of the organization first. Sally is a people pleaser in a people profession (academics, human resources, mental health, corporate training). She says yes to everyone and constantly works overtime to finish projects that often aren't even hers. Sally's wardrobe fills two closets and spans four dress sizes. It is a disorganized, disconnected collection of impulse purchases (many with tags) and clothes that don't fit. Her life strategy? Kill judgment in its tracks with kindness. For years, she has found little time to be kind to herself but a health scare has put her need for self-care front and center.

As far back as she can remember, Belle has played the role of nice girl. Parents, teachers, church leaders—she met everyone's expectations. An honor roll mainstay, Belle steered clear of the typical pitfalls of young adulthood. No drunken escapades for this girl. She was content to spend her free time with her youth group or family and preferred anonymous modest clothes (many sewed by her own mother) to the flashy styles favored by her peer group. After college, Belle married a wealthy man and forwent a career path to raise their two children. Twenty-five years later, newly divorced with two teenagers, Belle is about to enter the workforce for the first time. She isn't going to work because she needs the money: After spending her best years honoring a good girl image for a not so good man, Belle is hungry for a radical life change (within reason). Belle's closet is tidy, populated with a lifetime of sweater sets and literally nothing that reflects the liberated woman she is desperate to reveal.

Break the Dress Pattern

Women are unique, multidimensional creatures. Not every client falls squarely into a personality type but each shares a very real and specific impetus for change—and most don't recognize how self-image has shaped their narrative.

Like you, all of my clients are capable of, and deserve more: more happiness, more vitality, more mornings feeling like a bada**. For different reasons, they hide their best selves in cluttered closets, behind outdated clothes that reinforce old story lines.

Let's be real—a Ruthless Wardrobe Edit, strategic shopping skills and the Four Step Foolproof Outfit Formula won't mend years of self-denial, but when you leave your house looking every inch a digital era brand boss, you show up for work acting like one. Which is exactly the kick in the pantsuit you need to 10x your life from this day forward.

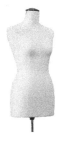

Are You a Michelle
or a Melania?

"Style is a way to say who you are without having to speak."
—Rachel Zoe

But First, Don and Barry

What about Don and Barry? This book isn't about Don and Barry,— or any Tom, Dick, or Harry. This book is a style guide for *you*, a smart, accomplished woman. Thus, this paragraph is the only ink I will dedicate to the male perspective on "suitable office attire." I am just going to come right out and say this: It does not matter what men think about how you should dress. This isn't your father's business world. If you actually work with male colleagues that expect you to look like a spinster, find solace in the fact that they will be dead soon. Time's up on the negative self-talk about what you think men think about your outfit.

Still grappling with the "but what if they don't take me seriously" question? No judgment, but no. Like all the others, this is a storyline crafted to keep your best, most stylish self at arm's length. You are a grown-up woman with good sense and an undisputed success record. You have earned the right to conduct an investor update in a sleek pencil skirt, meet a client for drinks in a form skimming silk blouse, or (heaven forbid) show a little toe cleavage in Italian made sling backs. Own the power.

The Work Uniform

Now that we've culled through the reasons you are ready to invest in your personal style and unpacked potential self-constructed roadblocks, it's time to get to the brass tacks on nailing your new look. First—don't get overwhelmed. Trust me. The goal of this book is to teach you a replicable method toward building a sustainable wardrobe you can rely on for the rest of your life. Because the majority of your life right now takes place at work, the core of this wardrobe is a work uniform.

Say what?

This coming from a girl who grew up kicking and screaming about the unrighteous conformity of Catholic school? If at 16 you told me my life's work would involve teaching women the value of a uniform, I'd tell you to shove it. But here we are.

I created a work uniform for the same reasons that powerful women across countless industries nail theirs: It fits, it flatters, it harmonizes with my lifestyle, allows me to feel stylish and put together daily and, with its common garment core and plentiful accessory options, it's endlessly versatile. Lastly, and perhaps the most satisfying element, during the panicked morning rush when I'm wrestling my six-year-old into his actual uniform, making breakfast and lunches, applying makeup (when can we outsource that?), and locating my husband's keys, I don't have to invest one extra minute to figuring out what to wear.

Best in Class

Your work uniform will be founded on several low hanging factors—your budget, body type, profession, and work culture, for example. Most of your uniform will be consistent, outfit after outfit. The goal is to create a reliable blueprint you can fall back on every day to look and feel authentic in clothes. That's the easy part.

The challenge comes when we seek to identify the very thing that has eluded you all of these years—the X-Factor. The X-Factor isn't a formula; it's the vibe that makes your uniform yours, a combination of nuance, texture, inspiration, and signature elements that add up to you. It can take seasons to refine the elements of your X-Factor but the first step in this process is to study the personal style of powerful women in our culture with that certain *je ne sais quoi*. Each of the iconic women below resonates with one of the Style Archetypes we will examine more deeply later in the book. Pay attention to the consistent elements they employ in their day-to-day outfit selections. What do their outfits say about their personality, responsibilities, and point of view?

Michelle Obama, Politics

The most outfit iconic First Lady since Jackie O., Michelle Obama's style is a hybrid of assessable yet aspirational femininity. Despite—or perhaps because of—her unique position as the first African American and the most educated first lady in presidential history, Michelle chose to dress in a manner relatable to her constituents and exemplified the quintessential post-millennium practice of mixing high/low to create an always unique perspective. Michelle embraced fashion and saw the power of her role in propelling (mostly) American designers. Save for her fallback looks—sleeveless sheath dresses by Chicago-bred designer Maria Pinto or fit-and-flare dresses with a bold print and waist belt—Michelle's uniform is the hardest to pin down, as she delighted in variety and experimentation. She was as comfortable in a J. Crew cardigan and pencil skirt as the iconic Jason Wu one-shouldered white gown she wore to the 2008 Inauguration. Michelle Obama enjoyed fashion for fashion's sake but she always looked comfortable, appropriate, and authentic in her outfit choices.

Style Profile: Michelle Obama, lawyer and former First Lady
    of the United States
Age: 54
Industry: Politics
Archetypes: Classically Chic, Editorial Eclectic
Uniform: Sleeveless sheath dress, cardigan, or knee-length
    fit-and-flare dress in bold print
Prints and Palette: Blue, yellow, color blocking, floral

X-Factor: Unpredictability, embellishment, bold colors and
prints, waist definition, athleticism

Melania Trump, Politics

While Michelle Obama opted to mix assessable elements into many
of her outfits, First Lady Melanie Trump's style is unapologetically
aspirational. A former fashion model, Melania looks every inch
the part in her uniform of four-inch Manolo Blahniks, European
designers, and a glamorous silhouette that emphasizes her height
and figure. Her preference for luxury aligns with the values of
the Trump brand and administration. Critics dismiss Melania
as a trophy wife turned reluctant First Lady but I suspect she
is smarter and more calculating than that. Who can forget the
fuchsia silk Gucci "Pussy Bow" blouse she wore to the 2016
debates in the wake of the "just grab them by the Gucci blouse"
controversy? Everyone assumed it was a daft oversight but I am not
so sure.

Style Profile: Melania Trump, First Lady of the United
States, former model
Age: 47
Industry: Politics
Archetypes: Full-on Glam, Classically Chic
Uniform: Slim pant or knee length sheath dress or pencil
skirt, blazer, cinched waist
Palette: Red and pink, cream and taupe

X-Factor: Enviable blowout, smoldering eyes, large belts, coat worn on shoulders

Sheryl Sandburg, Tech

In terms of assimilating your executive look to your work culture, Facebook COO and *Lean In* best-selling author, Sheryl Sandburg's work style is a study in contrast. While Facebook founder Mark Zuckerberg rarely wavers from his intentionally casual uniform of jeans, t-shirt, sneakers, and hoodie, COO Sheryl Sandburg is a power dresser. Her formal professional uniform has a minimalist sensibility that projects competence, seniority, and achievement. This sends a commanding message to her staff and the world at large: Facebook was founded by brilliant, boundary-crushing children, but I am the boss and we have a business to run.

Style Profile: Sheryl Sandburg, COO Facebook, author of *Lean In*; founder of LeanIn.org

Age: 48

Industry: Tech

Archetypes: Minimalist, Classically Chic

Uniform: Knee length, cap sleeve sheath dress, three-inch pumps, blazer or cardigan if necessary for photo or room temperature

Palette: Black, red, purple, cobalt blue,

X-Factor: Minimal makeup, classic bob, solid colors, matching pumps, strong arms

Donna Karan, Fashion

An undisputed pioneer in 1980s "power dressing," Donna Karan launched her definitive *Seven Easy Pieces* collection of business separates in 1985. Perhaps the first mainstream execution of a capsule wardrobe, Karan's collection was founded on the idea that, with the right garments, a woman could create a limitless wardrobe. The seven pieces featured in Karan's original collection (bodysuit, a versatile skirt, a pair of loose trousers, a tailored jacket, a cashmere sweater, and a white dress shirt) are indeed the foundation of many modern day capsule wardrobes, including my own.

Today, Karan's personal style embodies the versatile spirit of her original collection but more clearly reflects the philosophy of her current project Urban Zen, a combination apparel line and holistic wellness foundation. A devoted yogini, it's no surprise that Karan's Urban Zen line is made up of breathable separates designed to wear from yoga to cocktails: cashmere-silk leggings, twist front jersey tops, utilitarian jumpsuits, all with a global feel. Regardless of occasion, you will almost always find Karan swathed in a black cashmere scarf set off by an artisanal statement necklace likely picked up on one of her frequent travels.

> Style Profile: Donna Karan, fashion designer, philanthropist, and activist
> Age: 69
> Industry: Fashion, wellness
> Archetypes: Free Spirit, Minimalist

Uniform: All black everything with a bold accessory

Palette: Black, taupe

X-Factor: Fluid, draped fabrics, topknot or high ponytail, artisanal jewelry, yoga body

Anna Wintour, Fashion & Media

Nothing supports my thesis that your outfit choices send a much louder message than you realize better than Meryl Streep's famous adaptation of American Vogue editor Anna Wintour in the 2006 cult classic *The Devil Wears Prada*.

Miranda Priestly: 'This … stuff'? Oh. OK. I see. You think this has nothing to do with you. You go to your closet and you select … I don't know … that lumpy blue sweater, for instance because you're trying to tell the world that you take yourself too seriously to care about what you put on your back. But what you don't know is that that sweater is not just blue, it's not turquoise. It's not lapis. It's actually cerulean. And you're also blithely unaware of the fact that in 2002, **Oscar de la Renta** did a collection of cerulean gowns. And then I think it was **Yves Saint Laurent** … wasn't it who showed cerulean military jackets? I think we need a jacket here. And then cerulean quickly showed up in the collections of eight different designers. And then it, uh, filtered down through the department stores and then trickled on down into some tragic Casual Corner where you, no doubt, fished it out of some clearance bin. However, that blue represents millions of dollars and countless jobs and it's sort of comical how you think that you've made a choice that exempts you from the fashion industry when, in fact, you're wearing the sweater that was selected for you by the people in this room from a pile of stuff.

Streep's character, Miranda Priestly, delivers this biting line to her newly hired, fashion illiterate assistant Andy Sachs, played by Anne Hathaway, after she dismisses a pile of sweaters. It perfectly articulates the idea that whatever value you place on clothing, there is unseen depth to even the most surface level garment choice.

So how does real-life Anna Wintour, arguably the most influential figure in fashion history, dress herself to run American *Vogue*? But first, what Anna Wintour doesn't wear: Anything "trendy," head-to-toe black, nylon, and pants. Despite unlimited access to a universe of options, or perhaps because of it, Wintour relies on a consistent outfit formula of classic garments that she often re-wears, and of course, her signature pageboy bob haircut. Any given day will find her in a knee- or midi-length dress or skirt suit with a high neckline accented by a statement necklace and simple, often nude, leather sling backs. Wintour's work style is chic, timeless, and steadfast, just the anchor she needs to navigate the ever-morphing fashion cycle.

Style Profile: Anna Wintour, editor in chief, American *Vogue*
Age: 69
Industry: Fashion, media
Archetypes: Classically Chic, Editorial Eclectic

Uniform: Sleeveless dress or skirt suit with nipped waist,
  statement necklace, sling back pumps
Prints and Palette: Anything but black, Chanel tweed, bold
  floral, abstract, geometrics
X-Factor: Signature bob with bangs, large dark sunglasses
  (even indoors), svelte arms

Ellen DeGeneres, Entertainment & Media

Maybe it's the tomboy, sneaker-fanatic wannabe minimalist in
me—or the simple fact I've never met a sweater vest I didn't love—
but I heart Ellen DeGeneres' personal style. In a rotating wardrobe
of impeccably tailored menswear separates, she has nailed a pitch
perfect look that communicates her lifestyle, quirkiness, and sense
of humor. But the X-factor that makes Ellen's vibe so fresh? She
appears perennially comfortable in her clothes. Sure, I appreciate
Michelle Obama's malleability, Melania Trump's unapologetic
glamour, Sheryl Sandburg's consistency, Donna Karan's global ease
and Anna Wintour's failsafe chic but Ellen's take on professional
style is next level bada**. Why bust your back in sky-high pumps if
you can wear brogues?

Style Profile: Ellen DeGeneres, actor, comedian, television
  host, writer, producer, LGBT activist
Age: 60
Industry: Entertainment, media

Archetypes: Minimalist, athleisure

Uniform: Impeccably tailored menswear-inspired separates

Prints and Palette: Black, grey, denim, khaki, argyle, and pinstripe

X-Factor: Signature blonde pixie haircut, blazers, suiting separates with sneakers

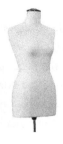

Chapter Three

The Lean Closet Model

"Creativity is just connecting things."
—Steve Jobs

The Fast and the Clueless

The most surprising similarity between every client closet I've encountered (and we're talking high earning, highly educated, professional women) is too many garments from Target. It's always the same story—they bought it because they were there and it was cute. They wore it once (maybe twice) and never since, because the sizing is off, the fabric feels funny, and now it's just hanging there. These items—and similarly "cheap, trendy, and cheerful" garments from fast fashion retailers make up the bulk of their closets and are the first to go to the donation pile.

Since the mid-1980s, popular culture has promoted the idea that very stylish women have very large closets. From Cher's remote-controlled rotating wardrobe in the 1995 cult classic *Clueless* to *Sex and the City's* Carrie Bradshaw famously realizing her Manolo Blahnik collection could have financed a down payment on her New York City apartment, if you came of age in the late 20th century, you probably equate endless clothing, jewelry, shoes, and bag options to the very fashionable.

Back in the 1990s, Cher and Carrie's fairytale closets were excessive and enviable—filled with coveted "it bags," Italian-made stilettos, and designer garments that most of us couldn't access or afford. Today, in the era of fast fashion, you don't need access or money to own way too many clothes—you just need a bigger closet. It's no wonder why the female buyer in every episode of House Hunters lists "walk-in closet" at the top of her non-negotiable list while her partner rolls their eyes. The difference between modern day walk-in closets and those of the cinematic icons we grew up with is that most of us aren't filling our closets with Dolce and Gabbana newspaper print dresses and Fred Segal collarless shirts. Our walk-in closets are stuffed with hundreds of inexpensive garments from ubiquitous retailers like Zara, Target, H&M, Ann Taylor, J. Crew Factory, Forever 21, GAP and Old Navy.

While it seems like the cost of everything has skyrocketed in the past 20 years, in actuality, the cost of cheap apparel has plummeted. In the past two decades, the number of garments consumed by global shoppers has increased 400 percent to 80 billion pieces of clothing a year (Eco-age). This growth has been fueled by fast fashion, a swift response system of clothing manufacturing designed to produce disposable clothes that mimic designer trends and push them to market in a matter of weeks.

There are so many "cute," cheap clothes in the stores you already frequent. Why would you invest the time in finding three $68 modal tee shirts when it's way more convenient to accumulate 20 $10 poly-rayon blend shirts from Target?

Why? Because research shows that women wear fast fashion purchases less than 5 times before they are discarded. There is nothing good about owning 20 poly-rayon tee-shirts. First of all, you do not need 20 tee shirts of any material. Second, rayon shrinks up to 10% in the wash (unless it has been treated with another synthetic finish to increase wet strength) so if you plan to wear those tee shirts to work under a blazer on a Friday, for instance, they will only retain an appropriate appearance for 1-2 washes before you relegate them to your sleep or workout drawer—and eventually the garbage—because you have better sense than to donate a used Mossimo top to Goodwill and they definitely don't absorb enough water to use as cleaning rags.

Now multiply that process by all the women in the world buying cheaply constructed clothes every single week from stores like H&M, Target, Zara, Old Navy—even entry level Nordstrom labels like BP—and you will get an idea of the impact a $10 tee shirt has on our environment.

As savvy, mature women, it's very easy to sit in judgment of the radical waste our economy produces in the era of fast fashion, and equally easy to absolve ourselves from that equation. But literally every closet I've ever encountered—the closets of lobbyists, orthopedic surgeons, network anchorwomen, and actresses—have all contained multiple "cute" garments bought in Target when "they just went in for one thing." The impulse shopping doesn't stop at the occasional big box store tee shirt. Closets of high six-figure-earning women all over Washington, DC are filled with poorly constructed poly-blend garments they don't even like or wear.

The Lean Closet Model

The answer to breaking the impulse shopping habit and conquering your closet chaos and the first step toward creating a functional wardrobe is found in a concept borrowed from the business world: the lean business model. The core idea of the lean business model, a term coined by the automotive industry in the late 2000s, is to maximize value while minimizing waste. A traditional lean business model includes practices like continuous improvement, relentless quality standards, and pitch perfect inventory levels. The goal is to cut wasteful spending, increase productivity, and maximize the customer experience. In my world we call this a capsule wardrobe.

The concept of capsule wardrobes is not new; it was popularized in the 1970s by Susie Faux, a British advertising executive. The daughter of tailors, Faux grew up with an appreciation of the impact a well-cut garment could have on a person's entire world view, inspiring them to feel and act with confidence. Later, working in the advertising industry, Faux was struck by the authority her male colleagues commanded in their suits and ties and sought to provide a similarly empowering resource for her female counterparts. In 1973, Faux opened Wardrobe, a boutique in London's West End positioned toward businesswomen with the goal of providing work attire that inspired confidence. She courted minimalist designer Jil Sander to the UK, using her aesthetic as the basis of her concept—a strong foundational wardrobe of well-made clothes that can be accented with accessories. She expanded on this concept in her 1980 book, *Wardrobe: Develop Your Style & Confidence*, in which she coined the phrase "capsule wardrobe." Today, women of every lifestyle have adopted a capsule wardrobe practice, but it was originally developed for career women like you who want to look great in their clothes but can't waste precious mental energy worrying about it.

In my practice, a capsule wardrobe acts as a blueprint to help you get dressed easily, look put together, and always feel good in your clothes. While there is no hard or fast rule to how many garments qualify as a capsule wardrobe, my seasonal capsules contain between 35—40 items, not including accessories. Each item is selected for versatility and to complement your lifestyle and body. The goal is to curate a lean closet in which everything fits, makes you feel fantastic, and can be worn in multiple ways. At the end of each season, your capsule is evaluated for productivity. Donate, gift, or consign under-performing items, store out of season apparel out of sight and then, with a plan and a purpose, shop to fill in the gaps. When properly refined over the course of a year, a capsule wardrobe will function exactly like a profitable business—minimal waste, maximum value, satisfied customer (you!).

Six Benefits of a Capsule Wardrobe

1. **Efficiency**—As you grow in years and responsibility, the time/money continuum becomes painfully apparent. When your closet contains only versatile garments that complement you, no time is wasted getting dressed and you can use that extra quality time to meditate or actually sit down to breakfast with your family.

2. **Cost savings**—When you break the impulse shopping cycle and adopt a seasonal shopping strategy, money once spent thoughtlessly throughout the year is spent intentionally during a finite window.

3. **Mindfulness**—The very act of acting intentionally conditions your brain toward mindfulness, which in time can curb impulsivity in other areas of your life. Perhaps you'll eliminate that second glass of wine.

4. **Creativity**—Steve Jobs aptly said: "Creativity is just connecting things." Inspired results come from the imaginative use of limited resources. When you've curated a wardrobe that works like a puzzle, every piece clicks together to paint a new stylish story daily, and there is tremendous satisfaction found in actually wearing all of your clothes.

5. **Confidence**—If I leave the house in ill-fitting clothes, I am acutely aware of it. *All. Day. Long.* I can't relax, or concentrate, or even listen to you. It's a problem. More than once, I went home in the middle of a work day to change out of a bad outfit. Who has time for that? When you leave the house confident in your outfit, you open up energy to obsess over something productive, like growing your client list.

6. **Control**—As a younger adult, I was totally laid back. But sometime between my career trajectory and raising small children, I became a basket case when faced with elements out of my control (like small children). At my breaking point, my wardrobe was one of those elements. Today, when everything else is chaos, I find tremendous peace in my closet, the one corner of my world under my complete and relentless control.

Lean Resources, Transformative Results

Like a lean business model, a capsule wardrobe is a proven method to maximize return (confidence) on minimal resources (time, money, clothes) and refine your product (personal style) in the process. As in business, transformative results require an upfront investment, in this case sweat equity, emotional commitment, and time. In culling your closet, you are likely to confront deep-seated issues you'd rather ignore. You may feel guilt and apprehension at the thought of chucking thousands of dollars of "perfectly good" clothes. After your initial Ruthless Wardrobe Edit, it may take several seasons of tweaking and experimentation to fully graduate from style inept to chic AF.

Will it be easy? No. Will it be worth it? Absolutely. If executed successfully, you will feel amazing in your clothes, all of the time. You will feel capable, powerful, and accomplished. As you clear the cluttered corners of your closet, your creativity will skyrocket because the process evokes a spiritual energy cleanse as well. Nature abhors a vacuum. What will the Universe fill into the space that used to house your $10 tee shirts? The possibilities are endless.

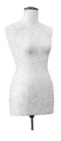

Chapter Four

The Ruthless Wardrobe Edit

"The space in which we live should be for the person we are becoming now, not for the person we were in the past."
—**Marie Kondō**, *The Life-Changing Magic of Tidying Up*

Manifest Destiny

By now you probably have a pretty good idea of the goal of this book—reduce your closet, cement your style, show up to work with off the charts confidence, close leads, drive sales. In business and in life, the key to success with any process is to visualize a successful end goal. Close your eyes and bring to mind a tidy, simplified closet. You can clearly see every garment, organized by color and category. All the hangers match. There is a dedicated space to display all of your handbags and shoes. Accessories are at eye level.

Imagine the weight of years of crap lifting from your shoulders. See yourself replacing awkward blouses and dated jeans with fresh garments that fit, flatter your body, and reflect your newly revealed personal style. Imagine a day in the near future when your most difficult morning decision is selecting a few accessories. See yourself getting dressed quickly because you already know what you are going to wear.

What is your mindset when you leave the house? Are you humming? Is it a warm, sun-dappled morning? Are the birds chirping?

If this sounds a little woo woo, it should. The Ruthless Wardrobe Edit is founded in the same principles as Feng Shui and Eastern wellness practices. This is about energy flow. A good closet has good energy. Before we can transform you into a style boss, you must first evolve your closet from source of stress to a sacred space filled with garments that, as Maria Kondo put it in her best-selling book *The Life-Changing Magic of Tidying Up*, "spark joy." This is how we'll get there.

Capsule Wardrobe Overview

- Reduce your closet to a manageable number of garments that fit your lifestyle. My seasonal capsule wardrobes range between 35—40 items. My entire wardrobe, which reflects my lifestyle as a full-time working mom in an office outside of Washington, DC, contains between 75-100 hanging items, total. If you live in a climate with little seasonal variation, your total clothing count should be between 60—75 garments

- Wear only the items in your seasonal capsule for three months
- Do not purchase any new fashion items during the first two months of the season
- Use the last month of the season to plan and purchase the items you'll need for the following season
- You can buy whatever you think you need for the next season but commit to staying consistent with your number and remove/store an equal item for anything new that you purchase
- Your 35—40 seasonal garments include:
  - Anything on a hanger in your primary closet
  - Short and long sleeve tee shirts and tops
  - Sweaters and cardigans
  - Denim, chinos, or similar
  - Lightweight jackets, blazers, fashion vests
- Your 35—40 seasonal garments *do not* include:
  - Undergarments and lingerie
  - Sleep or loungewear
  - Basic layering camisoles and tank tops
  - Hosiery
  - Active wear *specifically* for working out
  - Seasonal items like swimwear and cover ups, cold weather gear

- ○ Winter coats
- ○ Formal gowns
- ○ Accessories, jewelry, shoes, and handbags

Mise en Place!

Everything is easier when you have the right tools in one place. Before you start purging, assemble the following items:

- **1-2 garment racks**. These are invaluable to sort clothes as you purge. Additionally, I use a garment rack to stage outfits for the week, for an event, and to pack for trips. Plus they are great to have on hand for coats when you entertain.
- **100 matching huggable hangers**—Coordinating huggable hangers are imperative for eliminating visual distraction, the slim silhouette reduces closet space by at least 30 percent, and I am a big fan of measuring my wardrobe against 100 hangers. If I'm out of hangers, the gig is up!
- **2 Storage bins**—Use clear plastic bins for off-season foldable items or all items if you don't have a secondary closet, to collect donations, or to house items you are on the fence about purging out of sight.
- **3–5–4 large cardboard boxes and packing tape**—One for each pile: donation, consign, giveaway, and mend and an extra box for collecting mismatched hangers to recycle.
- **Full length mirror**—You can't tell if it looks good if you can't see your reflection.

- **Sharpie**—Mark boxes for storage, donation.
- **Notepad and pencil**—Record donations for tax purposes.

Do You Need a Practice Purge?

If at this point you are paralyzed at the thought of chucking most of your clothes, take a deep breath and consider easing into the process with a practice purge. Take a few hours to trim what I call "closet fat" and simply store it out of sight until you are ready to tackle the bulk of your closet. In my client work, I've identified five surefire places women store closet fat. You may find you make such a dent tackling these five specific categories that you are energized to finish the process.

Five Types of Closet Fat

1. **Off Season, Off Site**—Nearly 50 percent of closet clutter is visual distraction. If you have no reason to wear it right now, it shouldn't be hanging in front of you. Case in point: Off-season clothes. Start here: Remove every off-season item (clothes, outerwear, footwear, and accessories) and store in a clear bin out of sight or a secondary closet.
2. **The Fit Test**—If it doesn't fit, don't front. Box it up.
3. **Lifestyle Lapse**—Life, jobs, and circumstances are always changing. So often we hold on to garments that don't reflect our current lifestyle. If you once worked in a law office and now run a home-based consulting practice, you do not need multiple sets of suiting separates, especially if those

garments are more than five years old. Stay-at-home mom re-entering the work force? To the bin you go, LuLaRoe.

4. **Denim Deep Dive**—Let me guess. You have 25 pairs of dark wash skinny jeans, right? Pick your favorite three to five and pack away the rest.

5. **"But It Has Tags!"**—Be honest, it has tags because you bought it on impulse and it matches nothing or fits funny. Return it. Too late? Commit to wearing it in the next ten days or pack it up.

14-Day Love Your Look Challenge

After you've trimmed excess closet fat, commit to wearing as much of your remaining wardrobe as possible over the next two weeks. During that time, use the form below to record and rank your outfits every day. This exercise will help you identify what works, what doesn't, and what you need to fill the gaps. Maybe you'll decide to replace your entire wardrobe, maybe you'll find you already own quality clothes that fit, you just don't know how to style them. In many cases, my clients are missing items from this list of critical wardrobe connective tissue (ten neutral basics), which we will discuss in depth later in the book. Keep the ten neutral basics download handy as you evaluate the productivity of your wardrobe—take note if any of the items are missing or if you own them in the wrong colors.

Download the CTD Workbook for a 14-Day Love Your Look Challenge template:

https://tinyclosettonsofstyle.lpages.co/clothes-the-deal-toolkit

The Ruthless Wardrobe Edit

Whether you've jumped right ahead or spent several weeks easing into the Ruthless Wardrobe Edit, this is the part where we transform the energy of your closet forever. You may need to spread out this process up over several days. I recommend dedicating no more than five hours at a time to the Ruthless Wardrobe Edit. Drink plenty of water. It's a lot of physical work and you will also confront garments that hold years of energy, some of which might be difficult to process. If you can't get through it all in one session, stop, tidy up, and start again fresh tomorrow. Otherwise, you're likely to burn out and it may compromise your ability to finish all together.

Ready, Set— *Edit!*

Time needed: Up to five hours a session, perhaps over the course of several days

*If you started with a Practice Purge, skip this step

1. Assemble your garment rack near your primary closet
2. One by one, remove each garment from closet. Discard original hanger. Carefully inspect. Try on if necessary
3. Move anything that **does not fit**, is stained, or is in need of repair to appropriate bin*
4. Pack anything out of season neatly in storage bin or hang in secondary closet*
5. Evaluate everything left using only your intuition: *If you love it, you will know instantly.* Replace original hanger

with huggable hanger and return to closet. If you have any hesitation *at all* (don't worry about why), move it to the rack

6. Repeat this process until you fill your closet with 35-40 seasonal items that you love. This may take several rounds (and several racks).
7. Assure you have selected an adequate mix of pants, skirts, tops, sweaters, jackets
8. Store the out-of-season garments out of sight
9. Donate, resell, or give away the garments you moved to the rolling rack
10. Discard or recycle anything that is stained, beyond repair, or too worn to donate or sell

Keep or Toss?

I firmly maintain that if you have any hesitation *at all* about a garment, you do not need it in your life. But we are human—there is grey area—you will get stuck multiple times. Consider these questions when you can't make up your mind on whether something should stay or go:

- Do I feel great when I wear this?
- Do I feel guilty because it was expensive?
- Does it fit? Really? Like, right now
- Does it reflect who I am and what I do at this moment in my life?

- Is it dated? (Often applies to the cut and fit of denim and suiting separates you haven't worn in five plus years)
- Am I keeping this because I feel like I "should" (often applies to staples like white blouses or a black dress that you don't actually ever wear or feel like yourself while wearing)

Enjoy the Silence

Look at you! How do you feel now that you've trimmed your closet by 70 percent? Are you anxious, relieved, elated, sad? All normal. As you can see, there is still plenty of work ahead. But before you rush to Goodwill or dial up your local consignment or worse yet— go shopping—take the time to revel in your progress. The Ruthless Wardrobe Edit is the absolute hardest part of your upcoming style transformation. Take pride in the process. You've just wiped the palette. Now we can paint!

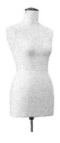

Chapter Five

Focus Group of One

"Great personal style is an extreme curiosity about yourself."
—Iris Apfel

Tell Me about Yourself

Recently, I was on a closet coaching call with a retired therapist trying to make sense of multiple closets overflowing with garments she never actually wears. After reviewing her closet pictures and talking about goals, we got to the personal style conversation. Her words: "Since I retired, I don't have any clothes for how I actually live. My closet is filled with either St. John suits or boho-style weekend clothes. And I don't wear either! I wear the ten garments that are draped on the back of chairs. I'm still buying blazers and I don't even go to an office. I'm either overdressed or I look like a hippie. I just want to see what I have so I can make an outfit that feels like me."

Sound familiar? She articulated the core problem most women face with their closets: They are filled with garments that don't reflect who they are or how they live their lives.

Like a lean business, which is constantly refining its product offering to eliminate waste and best serve the customer, a capsule wardrobe only works if it is refined to reflect its owner's needs. The reason your closet was a hodgepodge of unrelated parts is because it wasn't built on intentional investments—versatile clothes that fit your body, reflect your personal style, and were selected to dress you for what you actually do every day.

Before you dust off your Nordstrom card, it is imperative to identify who you are and figure out exactly what you need to buy. And I'm not just talking about specific types of garments, like layering camis or a nice silk blouse, I am talking about making intentional purchases that reflect a balance of your style influences and practical needs. It makes no sense to repopulate your closet with structured blazers if you are running a home-based consulting business. Which is why we first need to execute some consumer research—on you.

We will also evaluate your lifestyle—how much time you spend in an office, meeting clients, networking, with your kids, at cocktail parties—and make sure your wardrobe reflects an appropriate balance of clothes for each of those activities. Then we will identify your wardrobe palette and select the neutral colors that comprise the bulk of your wardrobe, which informs the accent colors you'll select to pair with them. Once we get all those details nailed down, we can shop to fill the gaps.

What Do You Actually Do All Day?

The bulk of your wardrobe should be grounded in the activities you engage in for the bulk of your time. As business professionals, one would assume that business attire represents the bulk of our wardrobe, but even in offices, there are levels of formality. Many of you are coaches or content creators that work mainly from behind your computer, but even if you hardly see anyone face-to-face, you still need to look good on videoconference and in pictures. I am always struck by how sloppy otherwise smart women appear on Zoom or Skype. Have you ever stopped to think how much time you spend on videoconference? Working from home doesn't excuse you from styling your hair or putting on makeup. Even if you are wearing pajama pants, do your clients a favor and make an effort from the top up.

One of my clients is a physical therapist. She spends most of her time in jeans, sneakers, and a polo top. She might have a super casual work environment but she is a professional—a medical professional. She owes it to herself and her clients to dress with a level of authority, even if that means sourcing the most flattering jeans we can find and a killer pair of sneakers.

As I mentioned earlier in the book, one of the reasons women own a lot of the wrong clothes is because they shop for stories they tell themselves about their lives, rather than their actual lives. Impulse shopping is a lot like emotional eating—you buy clothes that appeal to you in the moment, rationalizing that they will be perfect for a party, trip, or event that actually never happens.

On the same coaching call mentioned above, my retired therapist client told me about a gorgeous ball gown gathering dust in her basement cedar closet. "I bought it for a steal at Marshalls. It's exquisite: full length, black with a velvety trim. I bought it because I figured if I were ever invited to a Witches' Ball, it would be the perfect dress."

Prior to our call I didn't even know there was such a thing as a Witches' Ball—and now I want to go to one, too! But until I find the right coven, I'm not going to buy a dress. And even then, I'd want to know the dress code—is a dirt-cheap ball gown from an off-price retailer even appropriate for such a magical occasion?

My point is that a girl can dream—but she also needs most of her clothes to serve her real life, not her fantasy life.

Even if we spend the majority of our time working, an effective wardrobe is holistic, with a relative selection of options to dress us for weekends, leisure, and special events. Some occupations offer the opportunity for category crossover, which is yet another consideration in crafting a lean, yet well-rounded, capsule wardrobe filled with outfit ideas for every occasion.

We need to nail down exactly how much time you spend doing activities that resonate with the following lifestyle apparel categories and use that information, combined with your personal style influences, to shop for the best of what each has to offer.

Download the CTD Workbook for a Lifestyle Matrix worksheet: **https://tinyclosettonsofstyle.lpages.co/clothes-the-deal-toolkit**

Critique: Lifestyle Clothing Categories

Athleisure

Athleisure is a modern term to describe active-wear-inspired street clothes designed for ease of movement and elevated with on-trend details. Not to be confused with actual exercise clothing, athleisure garments are typically worn on weekends or for running errands. Some wellness and fitness professionals wear athleisure garments daily for work as do people across industries when they work from home or remotely.

Occupations:

- Yoga studio owner
- Fitness professional
- Physical therapist
- Graphic designer
- Etsy store owner
- Photographer

Fashion Casual

Fashion casual clothes can be dressed up or down with accessories. High/low style. Think: Denim, graphic tee shirts, camisoles, sweaters, tunics, tops, flat shoes, sandals, street sneakers, trendy accessories. A fashion casual outfit can transition from day to dinner with a heel and bag change. Fashion casual garments are typically worn on weekends for dates or dinner, to meet girlfriends, Casual

Friday for most offices, or day-to-day work style for creative or non-conventional industries.

Occupations:

- Creative industries—fashion, beauty, advertising, tech, entertainment
- Boutique owner
- Life coach
- Make-up artist
- Salon professional
- Blogger/influencer
- Personal stylist

Business Casual

Business casual attire is daily work wear for most office environments. Think: Suiting separates (but not worn together as suits), day dresses, dress pants, cardigans, sweaters, pumps, structured shoes and handbags, subtle or trendy accessories. Outside of the office, business casual garments are also appropriate for client lunches, presentations, or in-person meetings for people who work remotely, conservative weekend outfits, baby or wedding showers, school or religious programs.

Occupations:

- Most offices, regardless of industry
- Consultant

- Executive coach
- Academic
- Therapist

Business Formal

Business Formal attire is daily work wear for certain professionals and senior executives. Occasional work wear for most. Think: suits, a blazer and a blouse paired with skirt, dress pant, or structured work dress. Hosiery, pumps. Subtle accessories. Business formal clothes are also appropriate for job interviews, in court, and for funerals.

Occupations:

- Lawyer
- Doctor
- VP, SVP, CEO, CFO, CMO
- Politician
- Lobbyist

Cocktail

Cocktail attire refers to semi-formal event clothes mostly worn at night. Party clothes in classic silhouettes with interesting details like texture and/or embellishment that can be elevated with bold accessories. Think: little Black Dress, cocktail dress, sequined skirt, tuxedo blouse, silk camisole, fur vest, rhinestone statement earrings, metallic sandals, clutch. Cocktail attire is suitable for special occasions, the opera or ballet, holiday parties, charitable events, fundraisers, and recognition dinners. Regardless of occupation, every woman should have a few go-to pieces suitable for a special event should the occasion arise.

Occupations:

- Senior executive
- Public relations
- Event planner
- Entertainment
- Philanthropist

Something Changed?

"Lifestyle Lapse" is a term I coined for women who have recently made a major life change but haven't accounted for it in their closets or shopping habits.

My therapist client articulated this perfectly: "Since I retired, I don't have any clothes for how I actually live ... I'm still buying blazers and I don't even go to an office."

Many of your shopping habits are simply muscle memory. It makes perfect sense that my client would be drawn to suiting separates—that is how she shopped for the past 40 years! Clearly, though, those garments aren't serving her new life as an avid gardener who enjoys wine tastings with her husband on the weekend.

If you are having trouble identifying what ratio of clothing category garments you need represented in your wardrobe, ask yourself:

- Have I recently changed jobs or career direction?
- How often do I travel for work? For pleasure?
- Did I retire?
- Am I a student? Stay-at-home mom? Artist?
- Did I start a workout program or take up a new hobby?
- Have I moved to a different climate?
- Have I lost or gained several dress sizes?
- Am I a new mom?
- Am I newly single or newly committed?
- Is frequent dry cleaning in my schedule and/or budget?

Critique: Palette

The goal of the lean closet model is to ensure that most items in your wardrobe work together so you can create endless outfit options. To get the most value out of your capsule wardrobe, your palette should be as versatile as possible. So often I encounter clients who complain they have nothing to wear only to discover a closet full of lovely garments in a rainbow of accent colors and no neutral staples to connect them.

My seasonal capsules are typically 70 percent neutral, 30 percent color + print. It is critical to commit to a neutral palette before you shop to fill your wardrobe gaps. The majority of your wardrobe and all of your work uniform staples will need to be in complementary neutral colors so you can wear them together or separately paired with other pieces. These colors should also transcend most seasons.

You want your neutral palette to act as a blank canvas for every other color or print in your wardrobe. A neutral palette is determined by personal preference, sometimes occupation, and pragmatically by looking at the colors of shoes and clothes you already own.

At my job in the hair industry, it is a requirement for our salon professionals to wear black in salons, so out of respect, I wear black when I interface with them. I also really like black—it vibes with me. Unsurprisingly, most of my shoes are—you guessed it—black leather (or bright colors that pop against black clothing). In the winter, I supplement my mostly black neutral staples with grey. In addition to the year-round black staples assortment, in warmer months I supplement the palette with navy blue, because I think it looks softer against bright colors.

Neutral Palette

Select two to three neutrals to anchor your wardrobe palette. These can vary by season.

Ask Yourself:

- Can I create four to six outfits out of each garment in my current wardrobe?
- Do I have to wear a certain color for my job?
- Am I stain-prone?
- Does it get really hot where I live?
- What color are my shoes?

Neutral garments match most accent colors but not always each other. For example, I don't wear black with navy blue or brown, although some people do. But grey, cream, white, khaki, and nude match pretty much everything.

Your neutral palette can shift throughout the year but the majority should transcend seasons. In winter, you may pair dark grey and black staples with rich jewel tones and in summer, navy blue, light grey, and linen with pastels or punchy summer colors.

Neutral colors include: black, charcoal, grey, navy blue, olive, khaki, camel, tan, nude, beige, taupe, cream, ivory, white.

Falling back on the lean business philosophy of eliminating waste, it saves money on shoes and bags when you commit to a neutral palette. There is no need to invest in brown leather if you never wear staples that coordinate with brown. For this reason, I love nude shoes in summer and black shoes in winter—between those two leather staples I have a footwear option that matches every garment in my wardrobe.

Accent Palette

There is a school of thought that says skin tone determines which colors are "right" or "wrong" for you: Blue and greens complement cool-skinned complexions and warm-skinned women look better in brown, oranges, and yellow. I follow the mindset of the modern wine drinker—if you pick what you like, your instincts are right. Regardless of the accent colors you choose, it is critical that they work with your neutral palette. As you refine the core of your wardrobe—well-made neutral staples that fit, flatter, and reflect your lifestyle—you can supplement accent colors to experiment with trends and refresh the vibe of your wardrobe seasonally.

Ask Yourself:
- What colors am I drawn to?
- What colors am I wearing when people say, "That looks amazing on you!"
- What colors do I own but never seem to actually wear?

Pro Tips:
One way to land on an accent palette is to pull inspiration from a patterned garment you own and love, like a scarf or blouse. I've pulled seasonal palettes from scarves and even a pair of tennis shoes

Instead of selecting several accent colors, try two to four shades of the same color

Afraid of bold color? Incorporate pops of color via accessories

Download the CTD Workbook for a Neutral and Accent Pallet Planner:

https://tinyclosettonsofstyle.lpages.co/clothes-the-deal-toolkit

Ten Neutral Staples

I will never stop preaching about the importance of owning the right neutral staples.

My very first closet client, a 40-ish mom of two grade school children who runs a home-based recruiting business with her husband, expressed frustration at her inability to look pulled together. She really wanted to feel "casually stylish" when she walked her kids to school and for weekend dinners with friends. Even though her closet was filled with clothes, she was convinced she had no personal style because she could never seem to put together an outfit. What I found in her closet was dozens (and dozens and dozens) of unique garments, with interesting details, prints, and colors. Immediately I recognized her suburban Free Spirit style vibe. Her problem? Her wardrobe was a disjointed assortment of Free Spirit statement pieces and no neutral staples to connect them.

Neutral staples are the connective tissue of a functional wardrobe; these garments connect your prints, accent colors, and textures to create endless outfit combinations. Even though I recommend the same ten garments to every one of my clients, this is by no means a one-size-fits-all list. You will probably own a few each of the items in these clothing categories that are available in a range of budgets, sizes, colors, cuts, and fabrics—your ten neutral staples will reflect the mood of your lifestyle, body type, and personal style archetypes.

1. Tank, camisole, or shell
   - Layering essential
   - Wear alone for date night
   - Silk is versatile, season-less
2. Long or short sleeve top
   - Structured enough to dress up or down

- One neutral top is good, three are better
- Look for jersey, modal, or pima cotton

3. Blouse or collared shirt
   - Classic white is fail safe
   - Chambray for warmer months, travel
   - Look for silk georgette, cotton

4. Sweater
   - Layering essential
   - Wool or cashmere for cold weather
   - Cotton, linen, or knit blends for warm weather

5. Cardigan
   - Layering essential
   - Because: air conditioning
   - Look for same fabrics as sweater

6. Skirt
   - Pencil or A-line are the most versatile
   - Look for ponte for structure or viscose jersey for comfort
   - Should complement jacket style

7. Dress Pant
   - Go with dark: black, charcoal, navy
   - Proper fit is imperative—invest in a tailor
   - Look for virgin wool, ponte

8. Favorite Denim
   - Because: weekend
   - Invest—budget denim loses shape
   - Look for a denim/elastane blend for give

9. Dress
   - Go with dark: black, charcoal, navy
   - Versatile shape (sheath or A-line) that can be dressed up or down with accessories
   - Look for ponte, wool, crepe, jersey
10. Classic Jacket
    - Trench, blazer, leather moto, or denim—pick one in your style
    - Should pair with dress, skirt, and pants (but doesn't have to be the same color)
    - Invest!

Download the CTD Workbook for a 10 Neutral Staples Checklist:

https://tinyclosettonsofstyle.lpages.co/clothes-the-deal-toolkit

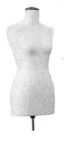

Chapter Six

Style Archetypes

> *"Fashions fade, style is eternal."*
> **—Yves Saint Laurent**

Defining Your Vibe

Until this point, we've focused on the tactical steps you can take to seal the foundation of your style evolution. The next part of this process is less straightforward; personal style is a nebulous concept. One thing is certain—you know great style when you see it. This is because style transcends clothing—it's a vibe. Style is the energy of multiple subtle elements that add up to a personal look with feeling. It takes time, energy, and self-realization to cultivate a wardrobe that feels 100 percent you. But here's the good news! Without realizing it, you've already spent years experimenting with trends, admiring stylish people, and collecting inspiration.

One of my clients, an international lobbyist frustrated because her closet was stocked with conservative suiting separates, contacted me to help her cultivate a weekend look. At 58 years old, she was convinced she had no stylistic point of view. When I looked through her closet I was floored (and surprised) by her vast collection of edgy rock and roll boots. Studs, leathers, fringe, suede, and leopard print—this woman's ankle boot collection rivaled Stevie Nicks! She explained that her husband (a therapist) played in a rock band on weekends. Challenge solved! We created a microcapsule of weekend looks around her boots, which not only reflected her personal style but also is perfectly aligned with her weekend life as a rock-and-roll wife.

Examine Style Archetypes

Boho, classic, vintage, preppy, edgy, downtown, romantic, glam, conservative, minimalist, trendy, beach, street, urban, athletic—the adjectives to describe style are infinite. In Chapter Three, we talked about modern business style icons and dissected the elements that shape their signature styles. While each of those women has a look that is distinct and recognizable, it's impossible to summarize their personal style with just one word. Like them, a range of styles will influence your ideal look.

I've categorized eight distinct style archetypes for you to reference when examining what attracts you. These archetypes are by no means meant for you to duplicate literally—these are not the only classifications of style nor will you find you are only drawn to one. Consider this list as a collection of ideas. Your signature style will come after you fine-tune a range of influences—but this is a useful place to start.

Style Archetype One: Classically Chic

The classically chic woman is a true professional. She is a lawyer, doctor, CEO, lobbyist, political candidate. This is the woman you bring to mind when you attempt to define chic—elegant, poised, put together and always exuding good taste. She relies on neutral colors, well-cut clothes, and classic silhouettes punctuated by simple, luxurious accessories. Disheveled is not in her vocabulary.

If classically chic were a city, it would be Paris.

Think: Coco Chanel, Audrey Hepburn, Jackie Onassis, and Carolyn Bessette-Kennedy

Classically Chic Wardrobe Staples:
- The perfect white button down
- Ankle pants
- Chanel style boucle jacket
- Breton stripe top
- Ballet flats or D'orsay pumps
- Diamond studs, Cartier tank watch, signet ring
- Hermes scarf
- Minimal make-up with a bold, red lip

Style Archetype Two: Editorial Eclectic

An editorially eclectic woman works in fashion or retail. Her experimental style is nurtured by access—to designers, buyers, samples, and showrooms. Heavily exposed to the workings of the industry, she's mastered the art of acting "as if" and always appears confident in her daily mix of prints, colors, textures, and influences. When it comes to the Editorial Eclectic archetype, standards of conventional dressing do not apply but somehow she manages to pull it off, leaving the rest of us to assume that she knows something we don't. This is a trend-driven archetype executed through styling. Her look is an interpretation of the premier designer aesthetic du jour assembled with actual high-end pieces (often on loan) supplemented with fast fashion (often disposable). Because of the transient nature of her wardrobe, her closet mainstays are neutral staples that she uses as the canvas for her sartorial fancy.

If Editorial Eclectic were a city it would be NYC or Milan, during fashion week.

Think: Leandra Medine, Jenna Lyons, Giovanna Battaglia, Anna Dello Russo, and Carrie Bradshaw

Editorial Eclectic Wardrobe Staples:
- Metallic midi skirt
- Perfectly imperfect draped tee shirt
- Raw hem or wide leg denim
- Oversized menswear blazer

- Gucci logo belt
- High/Low mix of arm candy: Cartier Juste un Clou bracelet, friendship bracelet made by her niece, round face watch, slim leather wrap cuff
- Statement shoe du jour

Style Archetype Three: Minimalist

The minimalist woman's aesthetic is deceptively simple but never unconsidered. Often works in architecture or the arts. Her look is one part androgynous, one-part athleisure, one-part sculpture, and almost always of a neutral palette. If she dabbles in color combinations, you can be sure it's black and white. Any design elements are expressed through interesting fabric cuts, like bold sleeves, origami folds, or monochromatic leather weave detail. A Minimalist often appears comfortable but she never reads casual; her vibe is crisp, cool, and sleek. Fit and tailoring are everything. The majority of her shoe collection is flat, she prefers slides or mules to pumps, and she isn't afraid to wear sleek white sneakers with a suit. Handbags are often black or cognac leather with minimal hardware and no logos. Accessories are typically sparse although she does love to set off a simple white shirtdress with a bold sculptural necklace in black wood, horn, or enamel.

If Minimalist were a city it would be Sydney or San Francisco

Think: Ellen DeGeneres, Angelina Jolie (now), Victoria Beckham, and Sophia Coppola

Minimalist Wardrobe Staples:

- Boxy white oversized button-down shirt
- Menswear inspired suiting separates, impeccably tailored
- High waist denim or paper bag tie pant
- White sneakers, brogues, or leather slide sandal
- Grey cashmere sweater
- Black dress pant
- Asymmetrical LBD
- Stack of thin gold rings

Style Archetype Four: Edgy

The edgy woman is all rock and roll. She works in music, photography, graphic design, or as a celebrity hair stylist. The edgy archetype is often described as an "off-duty-model" look, and Kate Moss certainly comes to mind when picturing this aesthetic. An anarchist at heart, her daily uniform of leather something (classic moto jacket, pencil skirt, or pants) paired with skinny denim, Chelsea boots, smudged eyeliner, and second day hair has a definitive slept-in quality. Unsurprisingly she loves studs, grommets, vintage band tee shirts, and anything that looks remotely tattered.

Edgy Essentials:

- Leather moto jacket
- Chelsea boots
- Slouchy vintage feel tee shirt
- Grommet or stud details

- Slim pants, leather or denim
- Sharp tailored blazer
- Second day hair
- Winged eyeliner

If Edgy were a city it would be London or Los Angeles

Think: Emmanuele Alt, Debbie Harry, Bianca Jagger, Kate Moss, Angelina Jolie (before)

Style Archetype Five: Free Spirit

Regardless of her industry or office environment, a free spirited woman is a gypsy at heart. Hers is a free-form, global aesthetic, she never wants to feel confined to a garment (or place), and as such, she moves with intention and romantic ease. She gravitates toward natural fibers like hemp, bamboo, linen, and cotton. She aims to know where her clothing originates and would rather support a line designed by a friend, retailed in a local boutique, or from a brand committed to fair trade and ethically sourced materials than shop for the newest trends. In step with her "all things with intention" mantra, her style is crafted with mementos from travel or items with history. She appreciates vintage and heirloom pieces. She gravitates toward earth-tone neutrals and plant-based dyes. Her prints of choice: batik, ikat, and similar global fabrics picked up on her journeys. There are always a handful of crystals in her pocket. While she appreciates the spirit of flowing, loose garments, she also understands that bare feet and flower fantasies are not appropriate for work and artfully balances roomy garments like wide leg palazzo pants with a fitted shell or pairs a slim pant with a loose tunic.

Free Spirit Essentials:
- Tunic top with slim leggings
- Ikat print scarf
- Belted maxi dress
- Long kimono
- Birkenstocks or braided gladiator sandals
- Ankle boots
- Vintage denim
- Beaded stone necklaces and bracelets
- If Free Spirit were a city, it would be Bali or Marrakesh
- Think: Stevie Nicks, Donna Karan, Talitha Getty, Catherine Baba

Style Archetype Six: Full-On Glam

When you see Full-On Glam you know it—even at her most casual (which is a stretch) this woman is a bombshell. Every inch of her look is considered, refined, and unapologetically alluring. The Full-On Glam archetype transcends clothing—this look is the full package and it doesn't come cheap. From her manicure, to her blowout, to her matching lingerie, a full-on glam gal puts in the effort. Where we choose practicality or comfort, this is a woman who is committed to her aesthetic. Unless she's in the gym (and you can believe she is in the gym), you will never see her in sneakers—the higher the heel, the better. She loves luxury, fur, diamonds, bling. Her skin is flawless, her teeth are sparkling white, her curves are unmistakable. She celebrates sex appeal and recognizes its power. Smart as a fox, she knows when to tone it down and when to turn it up.

Full-On Glam Essentials:
- 4" stilettos
- Silk blouse
- Pencil skirt
- Fur details
- Leopard print
- Sheer hosiery
- Impeccable grooming
- Red lips
- Enviable, voluminous blowout

If Full-On Glam were a city, it would be Miami.

Think: Sophia Lauren, Elizabeth Taylor, Sophia Vergara, Jennifer Lopez, Beyoncé, Melania Trump, Mariah Carey

Style Archetype Seven: Athleisure

The term "Athleisure" emerged a few years ago as a way to excuse ourselves for wearing yoga pants. Today, Athleisure isn't about looking like you just came from the gym—it's a mash-up style that melds ease of movement with sharp, tailored lines, a cool minimalist vibe and—most importantly—a dash of that certain *je ne sais quoi*. Athleisure may seem like an unlikely archetype for a professional style guide but if you consider the fitness industry generates 80 billion dollars annually in the US alone, you can see the value of nailing the look. The typical workday of fitness instructors, studio owners, and wellness coaches is spent active, either in the actual gym or virtually coaching clients about diet and lifestyle. Like lawyers or marketing executives, wellness professionals are considered the best in their field and they should show up looking the part. An Athleisure woman can run from client to gym without missing a beat. She has perfected the art of elevated yoga chic—an active base with interesting details like laser cuts or sheer calve panels under trend-forward top layers. Cut out sweaters, cardigans, Lululemon tights, with amazing street sneakers that do not for one second read track meet.

Athleisure Essentials:
- Lululemon Align™ leggings
- Street sneakers
- Modal sweatshirt with exposed back to highlight strappy bralette
- Tee shirt dress with side ruching
- Cocoon cardigan
- Fashion windbreaker
- Duffle
- Swell water bottle

Think: Jillian Michaels, Tracey Anderson

If Athleisure were a city, it would be Boulder, CO.

Style Archetype Eight: Americana

The Americana archetype is quintessentially East Coast. Collegiate style. Ralph Lauren. Polo, golf, tennis, sailing. An Americana gal was raised with a healthy love of green and pink and has never met a twin set or riding boot she didn't love. Forever appropriate, she dresses for the occasion but always with an eye to the weekend, preferably spent on the coast engaging in leisure sports. Her style is at once conservative and whimsical. Family heritage is paramount and you'll find a monogram on pretty much everything, from cable knit sweaters to cocktail napkins. Her signature items were likely inspired by her mother, and her mother before her: Barbour jacket, LL Bean Boat and Tote, Sperry Top Siders, Lily Pulitzer dresses. For work, she sticks to classically chic separates in navy blue or tweedy browns over black or greys. She loves a bright sheath dress and cardigan or a classic white button-down with dramatic oversized pearls or an impossibly high ruffled collar, tucked into impeccably tailored wider leg dress slacks.

Americana Essentials:
- Collared shirt under sweater
- Navy blue blazer with gold hardware
- Riding Boots

- Monogrammed everything
- Triple strand pearls
- Ferragamo kitten heels
- Seersucker or linen
- Lily Pulitzer dress
- Classic bob

Think: Martha Stewart, Laura Bush, CZ Guest, Cornelia Guest, Charlotte York

If Americana were a city it would be Nantucket, Washington, DC, Palm Beach, FL

Putting It All Together

Your style is more likely a combination of all the archetypes above than a head-to-toe copy of just one look. If you look closely, you'll see many of the archetypes naturally blend together, with elements that create bridges between references, for example: an edgy leather pant and slouchy tee shirt with a free-spirited floor-dusting kimono and floppy hat or an Americana collared shirt and crew neck sweater combo with classically chic ankle pants and ballet flats. As mature women, it may seem ridiculous to embody any of these looks, but trust me, there are elements of each archetype that will influence your accessory or fabric choices, whether or not you relate to the full body of work.

Download the CTD Workbook for a *What's My Style?* quiz: **https://tinyclosettonsofstyle.lpages.co/clothes-the-deal-toolkit**

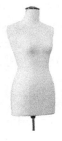

Chapter Seven

The Fool-Proof Four-Step Outfit Formula

"Accessories are like vitamins to fashion."
—Ann Dello Russo

The Art of Accessorizing

Capsule wardrobe success is all about versatility. Obviously, your garments need to coordinate but the *real* secret to creating a trillion outfits out of 37.5 pieces is the strength of your accessory game. Accessories are the critical difference between putting on clothes and rocking an outfit.

In my private Facebook group, I once conducted a style experiment where I wore essentially the same outfit every day for a week: Black J.Crew ankle pants and a black Vince boat neck long sleeve jersey tee-shirt. Each day I created a different look with accessories: Bright blue ballet flats and a white enamel statement necklace, cashmere cardigan with a Hermes scarf in my hair, arm full of bracelets and a knit sweater on top, killer pumps, and a sharp blazer. No one even noticed that my core outfit was the same two garments all week (hey, I washed the tee shirt!). That is the power of accessories.

If this seems intimidating, I get it. Accessorizing is an art. But girl, you've got this! You've already embraced your inner fashion stylist by creating a capsule wardrobe. Once you apply your obvious ingenuity to this easy accessorizing formula you'll be styling interesting, authentic outfits like you've been doing it for years.

Step One: Outfit Base

Your outfit base is simply the one to two garments that cover your nakedness (Think: Black J.Crew ankle pants and black Vince boat neck long sleeve tee shirt). You could definitely leave the house like this, but no one would call it stylish. This is simply the base layer of your look, which will be brought to life with layers and accessories in steps two through four. Some examples of typical outfit bases: dress pants + top; pencil skirt + blouse; dress; denim + sweater.

After a while, you will see that your work formula is simply a variation of the same core outfit bases, every day. This is why you'll want to think long and hard about what type of garments fit, flatter, and reflect your lifestyle before you invest in your Ten Neutral Staples selection. Your outfit bases are the workhorses of your wardrobe. They carry the weight of your personal style.

Before moving on to Step Two, consider your outfit base. Is it neutral? Colorful? Does it feature textural details or an intricate print? The complexity of your dress, romper, or top and bottom informs the complexity of the layer you'll add in Step Two. If there is a lot going on, keep the rest simple. If your base is a canvas-like blank—let's paint!

Step Two: Add a Layer

This is what fashion stylists and bloggers call the "third item:" an additional element that adds dimension via texture, color, or print. Think: cardigan, jacket, sweater, vest, or open chambray shirt. A general guideline is that the additional element can anchor the outfit even if you don't add a lot of additional accessories. With some outfits and especially when it's warm outside, you may not need another layer. But even in the middle of July, airports and offices are cool, so go ahead and grab that cardi or wrap.

Step Three: Make It Pop (Accessories)

Accessories are your capsule wardrobe's secret weapons; a simple necklace swap for fun earrings or a few savvy scarf-tying techniques can re-animate the same outfit base with a fresh perspective day after day, year after year.

Personal Jewelry

I believe a girl should own a few pieces of personal jewelry that she wears with everything. For me, it's a pave diamond disk (fifth anniversary gift) and my wedding bands. You may have a pair of diamond studs, a signet ring, or a delicate gold chain. Depending on the impact of your base and third layer, personal jewelry may be all you need. Should you decide to add additional jewelry, these items are delicate enough to layer over.

Costume Jewelry

This is where so many well-intentioned women fail the outfit challenge—loading on too many statements at once. When considering the following trend jewelry, select one per outfit: chandelier earrings, statement necklace, big cuff, or arm full of bracelets. Keep the rest of your jewelry minimal.

Whatever your jewelry choice, make sure it balances with the overall vibe of your outfit. White linen dress or gauzy bohemian skirt? Pile on the delicate layers. Pencil skirt with white button down? Pair it with chandelier earrings and a thin gold chain. Jewel tone sheath dress? Opt for a statement necklace and simple studs. Swingy pants and fitted tank top? Try a cuff and thin gold hoops.

Scarves

My Hermes silk twill scarf collection is the connective tissue that adheres my capsule wardrobe. My husband gave me my first Hermes scarf for my 30th birthday in 2007 but it wasn't until 2013 that I actually learned the one critical trick to tying the things. Inside that year's anniversary gift bag I discovered a sweet little orange box marked "Cartes A Nouer—Knotting Cards."

The Hermes Knotting Card deck taught me how to fashion scarves as belts, head wraps, neck ties, bows, bracelets—even halter tops—but the foundation for all of those styles was the one simple little folding trick I share in this video.

https://youtu.be/rS8Sgq1dEkI

Not every scarf needs to be Hermes but the optimal size for versatility is 36 x 36 and silk twill ties more elegantly than other materials.

If you are coveting an orange box, put one on your wish list! Birthday, Christmas, Hanukkah, Valentines, Mother's Day, Anniversary—all fantastic opportunities to elevate your accessory collection via luxury gift-getting. You just need to train the gift giver.

Everything Else
Some other ways to make your outfit pop:

- Belts
- Hair accessories
- Hosiery
- Watches
- Wraps
- Eyeglasses
- Hats

Signature Items

I love the idea of a style signature—an item or styling technique you employ in so many looks that it begins to define your perspective. Like my Hermes scarf collection, accessories are a wonderful opportunity to articulate a signature. Consider starting a collection of small luxury goods from a design house with an aesthetic you admire. Is there something you could pick up on all of your travels and incorporate into your wardrobe? Did you inherent your mother's collection of vintage brooches? Pin a cluster on a handbag! There really is no rule to what your signature should be except that it feels authentic to you.

Step Four: Out the Door (Shoes and Bags)

(Appropriately) Fancy Footwork

Like your jewelry, your footwear should complement, not compete with, the rest of your look. Bright pumps or exquisitely detailed stilettos could carry a neutral outfit on their own. Conversely, a bold print romper or an exquisitely beaded ball gown begs for simple shoes.

Above all, your shoes should fit the occasion. Walking up the Eiffel Tower in four-inch platform stilettos is not a good look. I've also witnessed the chicest woman in the room pair a formal gown with metallic flats. The secret to style is looking effortless. The secret to looking effortless is feeling comfortable.

Grab Your Bag

Thankfully we've moved away from the era of the "*it bag*," when every wannabe Carrie Bradshaw had to have a Fendi Baguette. Hey, I am all for beautiful bags (and I did own a Fendi Baguette), but much like my shoes (but probably more to do with having small children), these days I opt for practicality in purses. When selecting my handbag, I ask myself:

- Does it vibe with the outfit?
- Can I easily reach my stuff?
- Will I have children with me?
- Am I going on a date or out with friends?

Wrapping Up

You probably have plenty of accessories already; you just weren't sure how to style them. However, if you feel like you could use a few more pieces to round out your collection, hit up a thrift store. Seriously! I love thrifting for vintage bags, jewelry, and scarves. You can play around with different shapes; textures and colors without breaking the bank and you are guaranteed to find something completely unique.

Shopping Tip: For your best chance at scoring a treasure for cheap, scour thrift stores in wealthy neighborhoods.

Hopefully this basic to brilliant accessorizing formula helps you better visualize the elements of a well-styled outfit. As you get more comfortable with the process, you'll start to tweak the formula and break the "rules" to create a look that feels 100 percent you. (PS: There are no rules.)

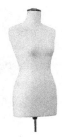

Chapter Eight

Your Grooming Game

"Grooming is the secret of real elegance. The best clothes, the most wonderful jewels, the most glamorous beauty don't count without good grooming."
—Christian Dior

Surely you've experienced the look-down. That not-so-obvious habit certain people have of evaluating your head to toe appearance with one swift swoop of their eyes. Your outfit takes up a huge percentage of this visual survey but your grooming habits are just as revealing— if not more so. The finest Chanel suit says less about a professional woman than chipped nails, sallow skin, and several weeks of root regrowth.

The Mind/Body Beauty Connection

Now, more than at any other time in your career, your effectiveness as a leader is hinged on proper self-care. Because stress is a way of life for high-level executives and entrepreneurs, your very lifestyle is in conflict with your general wellness. When the pressure is on especially thick, basic necessities like adequate nutrition, restful sleep, and moderate alcohol consumption are the first to go. At 30 you could burn the candle at both ends, but today the effects of your bad diet, lack of sleep, and that third glass of Pinot Noir are written all over your face—and it's aging you.

Like a fitness or diet program, the reasons why so many attempts at "wellness" fail is because they aren't sustainable—success requires extreme behavior and schedule shifts that just don't fit into the fabric of your lifestyle long-term. A simple yet profound concept: If you want something to work, make it easy.

A lean, functional closet, filled with versatile garments selected specifically to fit, flatter, and reflect your lifestyle lays the foundation for a daily personal style practice. All the work you've done throughout this book will make it easy to execute the principles on a daily basis.

How does the Lean Closet Model apply to your wellness goals? What can you tweak in your environment to assure your basic health needs are met? Better yet—what can you outsource?

Stress Symptom One: Diet Dilemmas

When the world is on your shoulders the last thing you want to think about is food groups but healthy hair and skin require nutrients to thrive. It's so easy to eat on the run, or grab a meal replacement bar, or worse, not eat anything at all until your stomach rumbles at 2 p.m. and you send your girl out for a deli sandwich and chips. If dieting is the way you manage stress, consider this: An extremely low-fat diet is directly linked to hair loss. Without protein, nails are brittle and hair breaks. Not enough vitamins and minerals? Could explain that bald spot.

Outsource: Meal Delivery

Foods that are high in antioxidants actually help slow down the aging process. Look for highly pigmented fruits and vegetables like blueberries, raspberries, and blackberries, which are the highest in antioxidants. Healthy fats found in avocados and nuts are also important for maintaining luster of hair and skin.

Meal delivery used to be a luxury reserved for Hollywood celebrities or people who live in New York City. No more! Thanks to the Internet, the market is flooded with affordable services that deliver prepared, frozen, or prepped superfoods to your home or office weekly for less than what you're paying at Whole Foods for groceries you never use. Some of my favorites:

- Daily Harvest (frozen super foods perfect for breakfast and lunch)
- Hello Fresh (family and kid friendly dinners, fresh ingredients)
- Purple Carrot (plant-based meals)

Stress Symptom Two: Lack of Sleep

Your body restores itself while you sleep but it can't do its job when stress and anxiety keep you up all night. Without the right amount of sleep, skin is sallow and hair doesn't have a chance to grow properly, which can lead to dull, lifeless locks. Lack of sleep can also affect your immune system and if your immune system is impacted, hair loss is one of the first symptoms.

Tweak: Nature Walk

Take a few minutes out of your day to walk outside and observe the natural world. Even in an urban environment there are seasonal shifts, birds in the sky, and clouds floating with the wind. Take note of what you hear, see and smell. **Studies have proven that walking in nature reduces rumination**, that pattern of repeated thoughts around a stressful situation. Getting out of your own head leads to better sleep.

Stress Symptom Three: Wine OClock

It's been a long day and you just want to take the edge off with a glass of wine. Soon your daily glass of wine turns to three and before you know it, you can't remember the last night you didn't have a drink. Alcohol also causes inflammation, which enlarges pores, making them oily and clogged. Finally, alcohol dries out your hair the same way it dehydrates your body and this can cause your hair to feel dry and brittle and break easily.

Tweak: Mindfulness Minute

Like all things in life, alcohol is fine in moderation. The key to shifting your wine intake from mandatory to moderate is mindfulness. Try to recognize the time of day or circumstances that lead to thoughts of drinking. This small act of mindfulness conditions your brain toward impulse control—and ultimately a night without wine.

Sweat Equity

If you don't have a solid fitness strategy already, it is time to start. Daily exercise helps increase oxygen in our bloodstream and improve circulation, which in turn greatly benefits your complexion. Most of us claim to not have the time to commit to fitness but seriously, if President Obama could find 20 minutes to work out most days of the week while running the free world, so can you. Unfortunately, you can't outsource exercise but you can throw money at the problem. Hire a trainer to meet you at your home or a gym close to your office, invest in some cute gym gear, and make sure to schedule your workouts like you would any important meeting. The easier you allow a routine to fit into the cadence of your life, the more likely you are to execute and stick to it.

For years I forced myself to make it to the gym three times a week. Regardless of whether I was tired, unmotivated, or just wanted to go to happy hour, I worked out dutifully—and hated every minute of it. Sure my body was toned and I benefited from the endorphins but I never looked forward to working out—

it was simply a non-negotiable chore like washing dishes. Then I discovered Baptiste yoga. With two small children, a full-time job, and a styling business, I've never had less free time in my life and yet I manage to practice an average of five times a week at Dancing Mind Yoga in Falls Church, VA. The studio is close to my home and office, so my practice fits neatly into my schedule. The DMY community feels like family, not a sweaty gym filled with meatheads and strangers. For all of these reasons, my yoga practice never feels like something I *must* do to maintain my figure—I look forward to the time I spend on my mat and more importantly—I don't obsess when my schedule shifts and I can't make it to a class. Yoga keeps my limbs long, my muscles strong, and my mind flexible. Find your yoga.

Best Face Forward——Skincare

Forever the product junky, I could write a blog post a week on all the enticingly-packaged lotions and potions on the market claiming to take a decade off your face but let's cut to the chase—there is no such thing as a facelift in a bottle. Yes, you absolutely need a skincare routine (more on that in a minute) but if you truly want to improve the appearance of your aging skin, you need to see an experienced dermatologist.

When our mothers were our age, the only solution to dramatically reverse the appearance of aging was a surgical facelift. God bless the cosmetic industry! For less than the cost of a high end skincare regimen and only 15 minutes in a dermatologist office, you can leave looking up to ten years younger. There are countless non-invasive procedures that will produce visible results but the most common, affordable, safe, and effective are Botox and Dermal Fillers.

Botox
Botox Cosmetic is an injected liquid used to treat frown lines, squint and smile lines, nasal crunch lines, and horizontal forehead wrinkles. By relaxing the underlying muscles, these lines become less deep.

After the injection, results are seen within 72 hours but it takes up to a week to see the full effect. Depending upon your metabolism rate, the results from one Botox session last between three to six months.

Botox has been used for over 20 years to treat thousands of patients. Botox is produced in a lab by a bacterium called "Clostridium botulinum." It has been purified under very strict, controlled conditions. Botox is made by Allergan, a company with a twenty-year history of making this product safely.

Botox injections are most commonly used for:

- Frown lines
- Lines around the eyes (crow's feet)
- Horizontal forehead lines
- Nasal scrunch or squint lines
- Lines on neck

Botox is also used in small amounts in a number of other areas on the face depending on the way your facial muscles work. It can raise the outer part of a sagging eyebrow, lift the corners of the mouth, and help to smooth out dimpled chins.

Botox is injected into the face using very thin needles. The entire procedure takes less than ten minutes, with plenty of breaks in between if you need them. In my opinion, waxing or threading my lip hurts more than Botox injections.

Depending upon where you live, Botox ranges in price between $250—$600, depending on how many areas are treated.

Dermal Fillers

Dermal fillers are produced under various brand names, the most common (as of 2018) being Juvederm and Restylane. Like Botox, dermal fillers address lines and wrinkles, but whereas Botox immobilizes muscles, dermal fillers plump lips and the hollow areas of the face.

Unlike Botox, which takes up to a week to see maximum effects, dermal fillers work immediately. Depending on the brand (Juvederm lasts longer) and the individual, Juvederm and Restylane can last up to 12 months before being completely absorbed by the body.

Juvederm and Restylane are both made from a naturally occurring molecule found in the body called hyaluronic acid, which, when injected, binds with water and expands to fill out and plump up the wrinkle from the inside.

Dermal fillers are most often used in the following areas:

- lines from the nose to the mouth (nasolabial fold)
- lines from the mouth to the chin (melomental fold)
- lines above the upper lip
- frown lines (best combined with Botox)
- lips for volume and definition
- to restore volume to cheekbones or cheeks
- in some situations, under the eyes
- to fill out the backs of the hands and make veins look less prominent

Dermal fillers are injected into the face and lips using small needles similar to those used to inject Botox. I think fillers hurt more than Botox, especially in the lips, but my dermatologist, Dr. Tina Alster of the Washington Institute of Dermatologic Laser Surgery in Washington, DC, always applies a topical numbing cream for 30 minutes before we start and has her assistant hold my hand and apply ice to the treated area immediately after each injection. All that said—the results are well worth any discomfort.

Restylane and Juvederm are usually priced per syringe. For example, filling out the nasolabial folds (the lines from the nose to the mouth) will take one or two syringes usually. One syringe will range from $450 to $750, depending on where you live.

Filler Up! But First

I cannot stress the importance of vetting a credible MD with years of cosmetic experience and great reviews before going under the needle.

Do not be tempted by the siren call of discount "Botox parties" and never allow anyone to inject anything in your precious *face* outside of a doctor's office. My first round of injectables was administered by an aesthetician in a strip mall medi-spa. The filler she used created hard balls in my cheeks that took weeks to dissolve and her Botox results were more Joker-like than the subtle "wow she looks rested" I enjoy at the hands of Dr. Tina.

Your Essential Skincare Routine

While truly transformative results only come from the hands of a dermatologist, a daily skincare regimen is necessary to protect skin from sun damage and maintain a healthy, hydrated appearance. It's easy to get overwhelmed at options (bless her syringe wielding heart, your dermatologist will try to sell you on her favorites) so follow these general guidelines to identify which products you actually need, when to use them, and which ones are worth an investment.

Morning

1. Face Wash—Save. Pick an option that works with your skin type, drugstore brands are fine.
2. Eye Cream—Spend. Look for a formula with caffeine to combat puffiness and amino acids to lock in moisture and kick-start collagen production. Use your ring finger to gently work a pea size serving from the inner corners of eyes and out toward your temples.

3. Moisturize—Save. It is *critical* you use a daily moisturizer with at least SPF 50 to protect your skin from aging and sun damage. Any SPF in your makeup is a bonus but it doesn't negate the need for sun protection in your day cream.

Night

1. Face Wash—Use the same product from morning routine. For the love of good skin—do not sleep in your makeup. Your skin cells regenerate at night and if your pores aren't clear, they clog. We've got enough to work against without worrying about blackheads (yuck!)

2. Exfoliate—Save. Use up to three times a week to buff dead skin cells and help costly serums absorb into skin better. Use a product that contains a mix of alpha hydroxy acids (AHAs) like lactic and glycolic acid to gently remove the top layer of your skin, which will even out discolorations.

3. Eye Cream—Use the same product from morning routine.

4. Serum—Spend. A serum is applied after cleansing but before moisturizing to deliver a potent shot of active ingredients directly into your skin. Look for a serum that addresses your specific concerns like wrinkles, brightness, acne, or hydration. Products that contain vitamin C, retinol, and salicylic acid will help to reduce discoloration and inflammation and unclog pores. If you have dry skin, check the label for vitamin E, glycolic acid, and hyaluronic acid, which provide additional moisture, increase elasticity,

and gently exfoliate. Pump a pea-size serving onto the back of your hand and use your ring finger to gently massage it into trouble spots.

5. Night Cream—Spend. Formulated to work with the body's natural healing cycle, night creams are generally richer than day creams and enriched with vitamins and antioxidants to help repair damage. Apply a dime-size amount to each cheek and massage into your entire face, neck, and chest.

Brass Beauty Tacks

Hair

Having spent my entire professional career in the salon industry, I know the value of great hair. I also know that most women would rather jump off a bridge than cut their hair short. To make matters worse, women with long hair hardly ever bother to style it on a daily basis, opting for a ponytail or hasty bun held in place by a large comb clip. This is not a hairstyle. This is lazy grooming and even if it's normalized behavior in your work environment, it doesn't convey authority and it definitely doesn't read chic.

There is a lot of talk about how a woman should wear her hair "at a certain age" but I don't care what length, color, or style you choose as long as it looks polished and considered. If you do not have the time or intention to execute (or outsource) a routine blowout, cut your hair a length you can style every day.

I've worn my hair in some version of a classic bob for most of my life. Thanks to my amazing stylist, Chris Houser at Salon Cielo Conn. Ave DC, it always looks fresh and hardly a day goes by that I am not complemented on my hair. It's a versatile cut that suits my face and hair texture but the chicest aspect of my signature hair is that I can blow dry and style it in less than ten minutes—so no matter how rushed my morning, I always look put together.

Color is as important as cut, especially at our age. This is not to say you shouldn't embrace your grey. White, silver, and platinum hair is incredibly sophisticated. In fact, as our hair starts to gray, our skin tones change as well, allowing these shades to complement the complexion. Note: This isn't permission to just say eff it and let your grey grow out. To maintain a professional appearance, it's critical to work with your stylist so she can gradually transition your hair to its natural color. An executive with half grey, half color-processed hair is not a good look.

If your hair isn't grey and you intend to keep it that way, make sure a salon professional retouches your color every six—eight weeks. Life is too short (and your time is too valuable) for botched boxed hair color.

From Miranda Priestly's platinum bob to real life Anna Wintour's blunt bangs (or fringe as we call it in the industry) your hairstyle is one of the easiest, most memorable ways to establish a signature look.

Cosmetics

Your years of experimenting with bold eye shadow, dramatic contouring, and a heavy makeup hand are over. And thank goodness! As we age, too much makeup actually makes us look older. If you are following a regular skincare routine, and especially if you've invested in Botox or fillers, you don't need a lot of makeup to look fresh and feminine. Some key tips:

- Start with a clean, well-moisturized face.
- Exfoliation is key to smooth makeup application, otherwise products will cling to dry patches, resulting in a ruddy complexion and cake-like makeup.
- Apply an illuminating BB or CC cream before foundation to add a youthful sheen to skin.
- Brighten the under eye: To life the eye area dramatically, create a reverse triangle under each eye, gently pressing concealer into the skin.
- Choose cream products over powder-based makeup. Powder settles into fine lines and enhances wrinkles, especially if you are prone to dry skin. Cream foundations, eye shadow, and blush will help to give your skin a smooth, even, and glowing appearance.
- Eyebrows thin with age, so you'll likely need a little color to make them pop. Opt for a shadow one shade darker than your hair color instead of a harsh pencil liner.

- Voluminous lashes are so much more alluring than elaborate eye shadow. Like eyebrows, eyelashes thin with age. Our instinct is to overcompensate with loads of mascara, which looks anything but natural. Instead, use an eyelash rejuvenator like Latisse® or Roden & Fields Lash Boost to add thickness and length. Better yet, invest in eyelash extensions—game changer.

- A creamy, neutral lip liner will keep your lip color in place and prevent feathering and bleeding of color around your lip line.

- Opt for a neutral palette over dark colors, glitter, and dramatic eye shadow.

Hands and Nails

Your hands get way more attention than you realize. Women love to talk with their hands! Keep a tube of fragrance-free hand lotion on your desk to maintain the appearance of soft, smooth skin. Even if you don't get regular manicures, it is important your nails are always neat—they should be clean, evenly filed and on the shorter side. A long, naked nail is not a good look. If you do get manicures, opt for neutral or classic colors, and assure polish is never chipped. Nail art, neon colors, glitter, or an extreme length is never appropriate for an executive—unless, of course, you work at OPI.

One of my clients is a clinical social worker and an advocate for the deaf and blind. When she is on stage and in meetings, she signs.

In her office practice, she prefers a minimal style of dress as to keep the focus on the client, not on her clothes. When we discussed the idea of a personal style signature, I suggested a signature nail polish—something bright, that radiates positivity, hope, and confidence. We landed on a cheery pinkish-orange shade that always makes her smile. Even though she prefers muted neutral tones for her clothing, her hands communicate the bright light of her spirit and vocation.

The Total Package

Grooming sends a strong message about attention to detail and general self-awareness, critical aspects that project authority. Considered hair, skin, makeup, and nails also create the canvas on which you layer personal style. Good grooming is as important as anything you wear to work—it is so critical, in fact, that I include a Total Package makeover in my premium executive style package. The renewed confidence that comes with a fresh face, flattering hairstyle, and the right make-up acts as a kick-start for the rest of our work together. Once my client feels put together, the idea she could also be stylish isn't such a stretch.

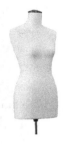

Chapter Nine

Clothes the Deal

> *"What is the difference between fashion and style?*
> *Fashion says 'Me, too,' and style, 'Only me.'"*
> **—Geraldine Stutz**

We started this journey exploring all the reasons you've neglected your self-image. By now, I hope you feel empowered to implement a plan to honor this very influential aspect of your life. Personal style isn't a magical power left to young people and celebrities—it's a skill set you are more than qualified to master.

The core idea of the capsule wardrobe is to maximize value while minimizing waste. Like a lean business, a capsule wardrobe is hinged on practices like continuous improvement, relentless quality standards, and pitch-perfect inventory levels. The goal is to curb impulse shopping, increase garment productivity, and maximize your outfit options. The capsule wardrobe is the system you'll adopt to streamline your closet and cement your personal style.

The state of your mind and body is arguably more important than clothes. Wellness practices like stress management and fitness set the stage for the healthy hair, nails, and skin. A healthy, impeccably groomed woman doesn't need an elaborate outfit to look completely put together. It is essential you address self-care to be an effective leader and a happy person, but seemingly small details like overdrawn eyebrows or chipped nail polish convey messages that could potentially undermine your authority.

Your daily look speaks volumes about competence, self-image, attention to detail, influences, and success level. An investment in your appearance yields a priceless return. When you feel good in your own skin, your confidence trickles down to shade your every interaction. Personal style isn't found shopping—it's an amalgamation of influences: Comfort, experiences, travel, relationships, texture, preference, and above all, confidence. People gravitate toward confidence. Confidence sells.

Will this process be simple? No. Will it be worth it? Absolutely. If executed successfully, you will feel amazing in your clothes—capable, powerful, and accomplished. As you clear the cluttered corners of your closet, your creativity will skyrocket. Nature abhors a vacuum. What will the Universe pour into the space that used to house ill-fitting blazers and out-of-date jeans? The possibilities are endless.

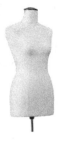

Chapter Ten

Conclusion

> *"I hire people brighter than me*
> *and then get out of their way."*
> **—Lee Iacocca**

When I attempt to explain the concept for my original blog and now my business—capsule wardrobes—I am met with equal parts intrigue and skepticism. Many assume I embraced "minimalism" to either save money or save the planet. While both of those are noble considerations, neither was the driving force.

I started this journey when confronted with a storage issue. Research for organizational solutions unearthed the capsule wardrobe movement. After eagerly inhaling every resource I could find, it was very clear that my problem wasn't storage, it was conspicuous consumption. I also realized I was sick of being held captive by my closet. Three years in, the process has improved my life in countless ways.

Had I not tackled my closet chaos and cleared its muddled energy, I'd have never started on the path that led to this book—and the opportunity to help women like you simplify their closets, cement their personal style, and make themselves feel amazing every day.

I am the living embodiment of the Tiny Closet, Tons of Style® philosophy, yes, but I am also a time-strapped mom with a nine-to-five job—in addition to my capsule wardrobe business. Style, beauty, and branding come very naturally to me. It's not work. It's easy. By 9 a.m. every weekday, I manage to dress, feed and prep two small children for school, *and* shower, execute full hair and makeup, style an original outfit, film a live Facebook video and Instagram Story about it, take nearly 50 iPhone outfit selfies, edit them down to one suitable for social sharing, drop kids off at various destinations, and get to my office on time (ish). Every day my co-workers marvel at how I manage to look so put together with so many responsibilities. The answer? Capsule wardrobe.

But you know what types of things I can't seem to execute? Laundry. Housework. Meal Prep. Play Dates. Organize my e-mail. Engage on Instagram. Program Pinterest. Design my own blog graphics. Update the press page on my website. Create a new lead magnet. Copy edit this book.

Why? Because I don't have any extra time! Even though I have the skill set and fortitude to complete these tasks on my own, I choose to pay other people to take care of them. Experts. Lovely people, friends really, who can apply time, focus, and experience to the to-dos that really must get done but that I don't have the bandwidth to complete. We are all happier people for it.

Yes, you can execute every step of my process on your own. I did it! Yes, it will be worth the time and money invested. Once you purge your closet and fill it with garments that fit, flatter, and reflect your preferences and lifestyle, you will look great, feel amazing, and own it at the office every day. Yes, this *must* happen. If not, your outlook will remain exactly as is—stuck, grumpy, tired, dejected. Not a good look.

But let's be real—do you have the time?

Would it be easier to hire an expert? Someone who lives and breathes style, beauty, and branding? A gal who can whip your closet, your clothes, and your outlook into shape in less than three days?

Let's talk.

xoxo

Jenn

Further Reading

Fierce Style by Christian Siriano

I Love Your Style: How to Define and Refine Your Personal Style by
    Amanda Brooks

Style A to Zoe by Rachel Zoe

*The Lucky Guide to Mastering Any Style: How to Wear Iconic Looks
    and Make Them Your Own* by Kim France and Andrea Linett

*The Life-Changing Magic of Tidying Up: The Japanese Art of
    Decluttering and Organizing* by Marie Kondo

Acknowledgments

A massive thank you to Christian Siriano for orchestrating so many magical fashion moments in my life: From #NYFW to my unforgettable wedding gown to your endorsement of this book—your creative spark continues to ignite my mine. I am so proud of you.

Thank you to my husband Matt for fueling my ambition, feeding me, and always telling me I'm pretty. I love you so much and I am very proud to be your wife. This book wouldn't be possible without my family: my father, Rick, the straw that stirs my greatness and my mother, Sylvia, for providing relentless creative tension and for teaching me to ask for forgiveness but never permission; to my sister, Emily, for humoring Matt when he calls and for being my very best friend; to my sisters Pamela and Margaret, whose admiration pushes me to be the person they assume I am; to my brother Ricky because he's smarter than all of us and not obsessed with proving it. To my Aunt Donna for always watching my videos and to my Grandmom, Joanna Yolanda Roberts, because I am her favorite.

Had it not been for Ada Pollo, Miss Fairy Dust herself, inviting me to present Tiny Closet Survival Guide to her highly exclusive Georgetown book club, I wouldn't have been reacquainted with Washingtonian journalist and *Crush* author Cathy Alter and she wouldn't have pushed me to apply for the Author Incubator program, who published this book. Talk about kismet! Later that same week, I reached out to the incredibly fabulous Master Certified Life Coach and Author Incubated writer Susan Hyatt for advice on the program. She gave me her blessing and I found a new source of empowered female inspiration in the process.

I couldn't have finished this process in nine weeks if it weren't for my friends' support: Crystal Street for keeping me real and appreciating a messy house, Pilar Bell for loving and laughing with me since 1983—and for lending me her Jimmy Choo bags which I sure hope I've returned by now. Thank you to Sergio Oehninger for that time in 2002 when, after I accepted a job in marketing, he expressed heartfelt concern that I'd never write again. How could I let you down? Thank you to the Bs: Joy Brock Tiani, Jennifer Caugh, Michelle Schaffer, and Michelle Wynn for their outstanding community leadership and for saving me from the drama of "Bs Chat" so I could concentrate on writing. My heart to Karina Giglio for scheduling early-2000s Cibu Marketing Updates so we could talk about boys and end up best friends and finally, so much love to Maurice Crittendon for always seeing me without, you know, actually seeing anything.

It's a funny dichotomy that my Tiny Closet, Tons of Style® side hustle would have never emerged without the confidence I gained under the leadership of my chic #AF mentor, Ann Ratner, who trusted me with her Cibu vision and gave this book her heartfelt blessing because she knows I am "capable of big things, love." I must also acknowledge the elephant in the Fun Room—if it weren't for Lisa Rieve, Josette Ashiru, and Nikki Posinski taking over all of the Cibu hard parts after I had Ashby, I wouldn't have been bored enough to start a capsule wardrobe movement. That said, I must send love to Kristin Lewandowski for listening to me b*** about boredom and everything else for the past five years. You are in my heart, always. My final Ratner Family shout is to my dear friend and fellow rabble-rouser David Jones, who always made me laugh and never introduced me to a video camera I didn't like.

Speaking of hair, Chris Houser of Salon Cielo Connecticut Avenue is responsible for one of the most impactful elements of my signature style—my forever-fresh razor cut bob and next level balayage color.

Like I said in the book, beauty starts from the inside out. My inside-out beauty secret is Baptiste yoga, which I practice dutifully with Paula Baake's team at Dancing Mind Yoga in Falls Church, Va. The DMY community is amazing and my practice keeps me sane, focused, and acutely aware that discomfort is temporary and 100% more manageable when you use your breath to "find the ease."

A big shout out to the Tiny Closet, Tons of Style Survival Guide community and all of my Tiny Closet University students, especially my ideal reader and biggest cheerleader, Kathy Gore Steele. This one's for you, loves! Be the bright and show me your outfits.

To the Morgan James Publishing team: Special thanks to David Hancock, CEO & Founder for believing in me and my message. To my Author Relations Manager, Margo Toulouse, thanks for making the process seamless and easy. Many more thanks to everyone else, but especially Jim Howard, Bethany Marshall, and Nickcole Watkins.

At long last, if it weren't for my desire to devote more time to my children: Custis, my first baby and the pup who taught me how to be a mommy; Andrew "AJ" James, my clever, creative, quick witted, and high-spirited boy; and Virginia Ashby, my mini-me and sassy fashion girl sidekick, I would have never written this book. I love you all so much. Don't make a mess. Thank you.

Be the bright,

Jenn

About the Author

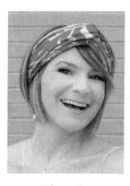

Branding and style expert Jenn Mapp Bressan is a mom, wife, lifetime fashion lover, reformed shopaholic, and capsule wardrobe convert. She aims to prove that closet size does not matter in matters of personal style.

But Jenn wasn't always so inspiring. She was once held captive by her closet; it was overflowing with clothes and overtaking her life. When she was single, Jenn shopped for sport. Then she started a family and bought a home. And while she had no business spending thousands of dollars a month on clothes, shopping became the way she dealt with all of her stressors.

At her breaking point, Jenn's wardrobe spanned four dress sizes and filled three closets. Where it once sparked joy and creativity,

Jenn's massive wardrobe now dulled her sparkly aura. That's when Jenn had an epiphany—the things she owned actually owned her.

She ruthlessly ripped through her wardrobe and purged anything she didn't truly love. When finished, Jenn's closet contained only 37.5 core garments. After a lifetime of shopping, Jenn never felt as stylish as when she gave away most of her wardrobe.

Now a big believer in capsule wardrobes, Jenn rehabs closet junkies such as WJLA's Alison Starling and The Walking Dead's Ann Mahoney by applying her "Tiny Closet, Tons of Style®" editing philosophy to their wardrobes. In 2017, her business was honored in Washingtonian Magazine's annual Best of DC issue.

Website: MappCraft | Tiny Closet, Tons of Style®
Facebook: MappCraft | Tiny Closet Survival Guide
Instagram: @TinyClosetTonsofStyle
Email: jenn.mapp@mappcraft.com

Thank You

Dear Reader,

Thank you so much for buying my book.

I wish you amazing success on your journey to conquer closet chaos and cement your personal style. As a token of my gratitude, please accept your FREE gift (**https://tinyclosettonsofstyle.lpages. co/clothes-the-deal-toolkit**), a supplemental tool kit created to help you execute the key steps I outlined in this book. These are just a few of the actual materials I use with both real life and virtual closet coaching clients.

The Clothes the Deal Tool Kit includes:

- Lifestyle Matrix Worksheet
- Style Archetype Quiz
- 14 Day Love Your Look Challenge
- Neutral and Accent Palette Planner

- 10 Neutral Staples Checklist
- Free Style Strategy call with Jenn

And if there's anything else I can do to help you, please email me at jennmapp@mappcraft.com

Sincerely,
Jenn Mapp Bressan
Founder, MappCraft | Tiny Closet, Tons of Style

Visit **https://tinyclosettonsofstyle.lpages.co/clothes-the-deal-toolkit** for your free gift, to schedule a style strategy session, or for more information on my personal style and closet coaching services.

CPSIA information can be obtained
at www.ICGtesting.com
Printed in the USA
BVHW051827100619
550597BV00003B/4/P